An easy-to-follow and very effective weight loss approach

At last…The real ***weight loss*** book, for real people like you and me!

(Lose weight forever *without going on a diet)*

S P Grainger

First published by SPG Publications in 2016

ISBN: 978-0-9954906-2-8

Disclaimer: The weight loss approach outlined in this book is based on the opinions, experience and conclusions of the author. Please note that the author is not a scientist or medical practitioner. The approach is based upon the conclusions of the author as he conducted his own personal research, and successfully applied the results to his own weight loss journey. This worked for the author; however, the onus is on the reader to make sure that it is suitable him/her. The author and publisher accept no liability arising directly or indirectly from the use or application of any information contained in this book.

Published by:
SPG Publications
PO Box 367
BANGOR
BT20 9FG
Email: spg.publications@gmail.com

Dedication

This book is dedicated to:

My late Mum and Dad.

My family

Thank you

A very special thanks Kathleen Bates, author of the inspirational book *Joyful Witness* (tslbooks.uk). Impressed by my weight loss, Kathleen encouraged me to write this book and kindly offered to edit the text.

A big thank you to Glenn Hanna for his help with the cover design.

Contents

Part One

WHAT YOU NEED TO KNOW ABOUT LOSING WEIGHT AND KEEPING ITOFF FOREVER - WITHOUT GOING ON A DIET

Chapter 1

The proven-by-experience way to lose weight forever – without diets.

This was me before and after weight loss.

Before weight loss:

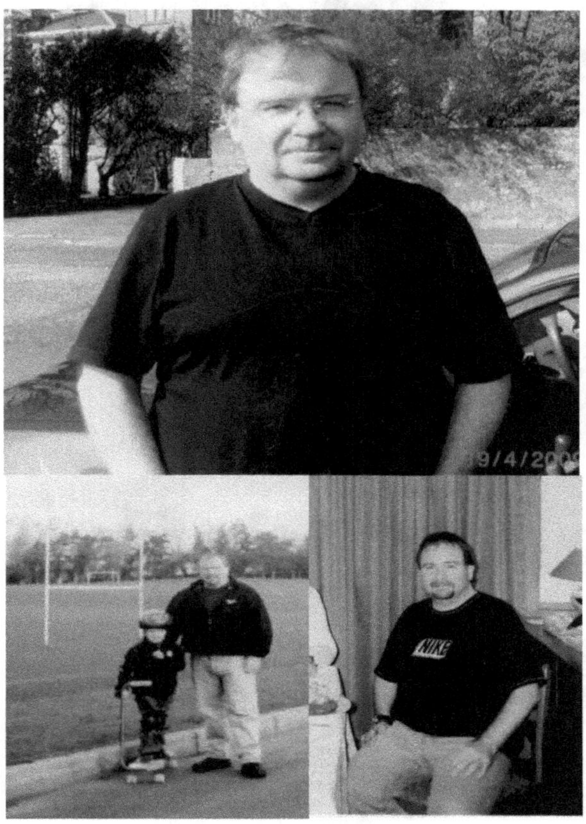

After weight loss (I lost 4½ stone/63 pounds):

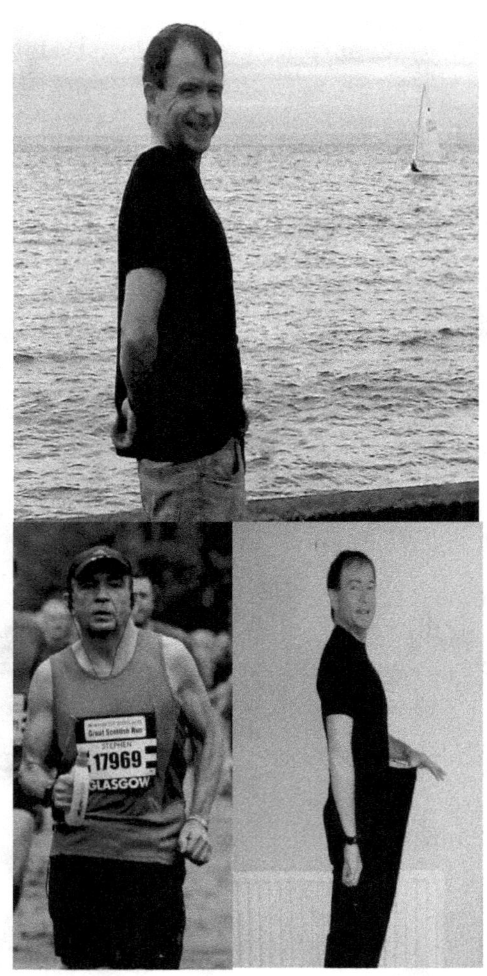

I am sharing with you how I lost the weight without 'diets' or gimmicks because I want to help you achieve the healthy weight that you really want.

Diets do not work! I know this for a fact.

For years I had tried and failed to lose weight with all sorts of diets. Thankfully I finally discovered the true secret to losing weight and keeping it off permanently, and found that it is actually *easier* than going on a 'diet'!

This book started out as my journal where I recorded my weight loss and fitness levels. At the start of this journey I was overweight (four and a half stone/sixty three pounds in fact) and an unfit 'couch potato'.

Now I am four and a half stone *lighter* and feel fit and much healthier.

How did I achieve this?

I achieved this when I stopped *going on diets* and *counting calories*!

Diets didn't work for me!

I found a better, more effective way to lose weight in a straightforward and natural way. The fact that you are reading this book means that you are in the same place as I was. You are probably just like me – facing the same struggle with your weight.

Are you unhappy with your current weight, afraid to step on the scales?

I couldn't sustain diets, count calories or use willpower. Does this sound familiar? If the answer is yes, you are just the same as me!

I know what it is to be overweight and unfit and long to be a healthy weight and full of energy. This is why I have expanded the record of my own weight loss journey and turned it into this book. I want to help you!

There are many books and programmes available out there claiming that you can achieve the body of your dreams. The diet and weight loss industry is worth millions, and thousands of overweight people at this very moment are currently following some diet programme or other. I know, because I was one of them! But in fact, every time I tried to lose weight I actually ended up gaining weight became increasingly *heavier*!

The good news is that I eventually discovered the best way to achieve my ideal weight, and this book is a record of how I at last succeeded in getting rid of all those unwanted pounds.

If you follow the procedures in the following pages you can lose weight and become fitter in a real, natural and *permanent* way.

You will be amazed how you can achieve this without punishing yourself with strict diets and difficult fitness regimes.

No gimmicks, no endless calorie counting; no torturing yourself with strict diets with boring food.

What qualifies me to say this? Easy answer – I am the same as you, and this approach worked for me. If it worked for me, it can work for you.

You may have read diet books before, and may think this is just another diet book. *No it is not!* You may also think that this is another gimmick or, even worse, some sort of weird alternative therapy approach to weight loss.

Please rest assured that this is no weird gimmick!

Furthermore, it is not a 'diet' or some sort of alternative therapy.

Rather, it is a process to lose weight based on how you and I have been created and designed to eat and manage weight. It is the natural way, or 'Nature's way' may be a more accurate description.

It is a process that is more effective than diets. In fact it will set you free from the misery of being a slave to diets. I say this because I know what it is like to follow diets – it is miserable and it does feel like being a slave to what we can and can't eat, and always counting calories.

Then there is the guilt of eating too many calories, or the wrong type of food. This guilt is magnified when we eat a food item that we actually really enjoy.

When we finally give up trying to follow the diet, which inevitably we will do, we then feel down and our self-esteem takes a battering because we have failed to lose the weight and keep it off.

In fact, I always became fatter after a diet, and so do most people who try to follow a diet. *There is a reason for this* and I will go into this in greater detail later in the book.

Please read this book with an open mind. I can say with confidence that the weight loss and fitness principles outlined can work for you, as they have worked for me.

I am living proof that this weight loss approach works. I am just the same as you, so it can also work for you – if you trust and follow the key principles outlined in the following pages.

<u>Before and after</u>

My life really was 'before and after' as a result of my weight loss in more ways than one. I have regained a quality of life and health benefits that I have not enjoyed since my mid-twenties, before I started my slide into the bad eating habits that eventually led me to become overweight.

I was so unhealthy, unfit and overweight that my health was really going downhill fast. I was on three tablets a day for high blood pressure and high cholesterol.

These problems were a direct result of my lifestyle. I can now say that the *weight loss approach* I followed, and which I now describe in this book, was so successful that my blood pressure and cholesterol levels have dropped (dramatically) to healthy ones. I no longer take any of the tablets for my lifestyle-related problems.

<u>**N.B.**</u> My doctor monitored my weight loss and fitness programme and only took me off the pills when he was sure that I no longer needed them. I still keep in contact with my doctor who will continue to monitor my blood pressure, cholesterol, etc. Remember, you should also let

your doctor monitor your weight loss and fitness programme. ***Only stop medication on the advice of your doctor!***

I have been set free from the 'prison' of my weight loss – no longer self-conscious about my size. No longer restricted in the activities I can do because of the restrictions resulting from my fitness levels (my wheezing, puffing and panting when I climb stairs or walk up a hill are over). I used to struggle with my extremely low energy levels and used to sit down exhausted when I came home from work. Now my energy levels are very high and I have an active life.

Please note that I am not promising you that you will no longer need medication; however, my health has greatly improved as a result of my weight loss and fitness journey.

I have also developed a high level of fitness in addition to my weight loss. As with weight loss, I discovered the best way to fitness is not to punish yourself in a gym! I will talk more about how you can also become fitter in a way that you will be able to achieve and that will become a real and natural part of your life. I was a 'couch potato' who moved from this low level of fitness to being able to run a half-marathon. Furthermore, I have just qualified as a Fitness Instructor – something I would have considered impossible before.

I used to take my young son to the park to play football with him, as Dads do. We did have many great times together and I will always treasure these special, happy memories. However, one of my biggest regrets is how my overweight and unfit body was unable to give him the higher quality football experience that he deserved. If only I had possessed the healthy weight and fitness levels that I now have!

The increased fitness level I achieved and refer to really is one of the ‘before and after’ benefits of my weight loss programme.

I was fit and active up to my mid-twenties; however, this declined as I became more and more overweight. I really had thought that my fitness days were behind me and certainly didn’t imagine that I would be able to reach my present level.

You may not want or be able to take up running or become a Fitness Instructor; however, this doesn’t really matter, as you are a unique individual, and you will find that the natural way of losing weight outlined in this book will be unique to you, as will the fitness benefits.

As long as you do engage in some sort of fitness activity for the benefit of your health, the way you do this will be appropriate to your age, medical conditions, current fitness levels, etc.

Remember, you are looking to achieve the ideal healthy weight for **you**, which will be different from that of your friends, family, work colleagues and just about anybody else that you will come across.

Why is this? Because you are unique in terms of your genetics, body composition, bone structure, etc. To lose weight in the way that is natural and lasting, you must tune into how *you* have been genetically programmed to eat, and re-educate your eating habits to be consistent with your individual genetic programming.

It is my sincere desire to help you change your life in the way that I have done. Remember: if I can do it, so can you!

Chapter 2

Why diets do not work

Lose 2 stone in 2 weeks!
Drop a dress size in 3 weeks!
Get six-pack abs and lose your beer belly in 4 weeks!

How familiar are these kinds of claims as we read newspapers and magazines, or watch TV?

Phrases like these grab our attention because we all want them to be true. If only they were true! Unfortunately, the bad news is not what we want to hear – these claims are completely false. I am going to tell you an important truth which I discovered: after trying so hard to lose it, I had actually *gained* weight! Why did this happen?

I will be making reference throughout this book to the fact that I decided to conduct my *own* research into why diets didn't work for me. I looked at the eating pattern of the naturally-healthy weight person to attempt to work out why they maintained a healthy weight without all of the diet and calorie-counting burden and constant misery of being 'on a diet'.

I was now really excited about my discoveries – especially as I was steadily losing weight in a natural way.

My excitement at the weight loss created an enthusiasm to look deeper into *why* the approach I was now following was working so well - in complete contrast to all of my previous failed 'diets' and 'diet programmes'.

I decided to look at the ***science*** behind why the 'natural' approach was working. I made some very interesting discoveries.

One of the most significant facts that I came to understand is actually fundamental to understanding why diets don't work: *when you diet you are actually going against Nature*.

Why are we going against Nature?

You are genetically programmed **not** to achieve weight loss by dieting.

If you attempt to lose weight by going on a diet, you are actually going against Nature because you have been designed to survive – this instinct is fundamental to all of your genetic programming – *you cannot go against this*.

You need to eat to survive. Sadly, human beings do not always get enough to eat. We in the West have become used to having plenty of food. This was not always the case, as a shortage of food was the worry faced by many of our grandparents and great-grandparents. Many people throughout the world today do not have enough food.

Human beings are remarkable in the way that they have been designed, because we have a self-defence mechanism against starving to death and of *making do* if there is a drop in the amount of food available.

It works like this:

Your body gets used to a certain amount of regular food intake. This is the amount you have 'programmed' your body to expect. If your body is suddenly subjected to a drop in food intake, your subconscious self-defence mechanisms will automatically put your system into 'starvation mode.'

If you stop eating the way you are used to, (conditioned by habit), your brain will be tricked into sending the signal to your system that you are in a famine situation and that food is in short supply. Your brain will seek to survive on the food available – until you have access again to the level of food intake your body has become used to expect (conditioned by upbringing, bad habits, emotional eating, etc).

Your metabolism will slow down and the reduced amount of food will be broken down and digested more slowly by your body because it is now in self-defence mode.

The reason for this is that the body is making sure that the limited food available is used for your continued survival in this 'famine' situation. Your brain has put your body into 'starvation' mode.

Your body will also 'borrow' from your fat reserves, with the result that you will lose weight – possibly a *lot* of weight in a very short period of time. However, this is only a *temporary* weight loss, brought about by the body defending itself from the effects of the perceived lack of food.

Remember, the body mechanism cannot tell the difference between a real shortage of food and a shortage brought about by a self-inflicted food shortage – a diet.

This is your genetic programming – *you cannot change this fact of Nature.*

Once you come off whatever diet programme you had been following, (and over 90 percent of people *do* come off the diet programme), your genetic self-defence programme will believe that the threat of starvation is now over. It will now tell your body to make up for the lost food intake lost during the 'famine'.

Because once the body believes that the famine is over it will demand that you go back to the level of food it was used to before the famine (the amount of food you conditioned your body to expect through overeating, habit eating, emotional eating, etc).

Your metabolism will speed up and you will be bombarded by signals from your body to fill it with food. You will not be able to resist these signals by willpower – your genetic programming is too strong for you to resist!

Remember the fat reserves that your 'slowed down' metabolism borrowed from during the 'famine'? The bad news is your body will want to replace the fat borrowed back to the level it is used to having (remember, you have conditioned your body to expect a certain level of food).

The subconscious self-defence anti-starvation defence systems in your brain cannot distinguish between a famine or crash diet.

Result of this: you will put on the weight, often with interest (i.e., you will often put on *more* weight). I know because I always used to put on weight after a diet.

Solution: you must get your body to get used to expecting less food as the 'norm'. In other words you must ***change and re-educate your eating habits.***

The good news is this process of changing your eating habits is easier than 'punishing' yourself by 'going on a diet'.

How you eat is a habit into which you have been conditioned. Not one of us was born to desire a big double cheeseburger with extra fries! Remember, these unhealthy eating habits are drummed into us by society and advertising, etc.

We also overeat because of emotional pressure and pure *bad habit*.

Our eating patterns and amount eaten form a *habit*. As long as you are used to eating at a certain level, your body will become used to that amount and expect and desire to eat at that level – your body has been conditioned to desire that amount.

You cannot stop yourself; as already stated, you are *genetically programmed to resist diets!*

Diets cannot and will not work for the majority of people – end of story!

What do I mean by *re-educating your eating habits?* In other words, *change how your brain tells your body how much food it needs to eat*. When your body gets used to expecting less food, you will have found the secret of natural, permanent weight loss.

Great news! This is not as hard as you think – it is easier than dieting and produces permanent results.

Chapter 3

How did I do it?

The first major breakthrough in my journey to permanent weight loss and good fitness levels was when I realised that all of the popular and commonly advocated diet programmes and 'received wisdom' were actually *wrong*.

Diets, counting calories, strict eating patterns, etc, just did not work long-term for me. I could not stick to them and I always became fatter after the initial weight loss.

Why was this?

My willpower was useless and I just could not get the weight loss I desired. I also longed to be fit; however, because I was so overweight, I could not do the exercises at the levels I needed and longed to do – I just didn't have the energy. I did walk the dog and walk to the shops, but this was not enough and was made meaningless by the amount and types of food I was scoffing. I decided to look at the whole area of weight loss and fitness in a completely different way.

<u>The naturally healthy-weight person?</u>

Have you ever noticed that person in your family, group of friends or work place who just never put on weight? They appear to effortlessly maintain a healthy-weight; however, they don't obsess about food or punish themselves with harsh and strict diets. These naturally healthy-weight people don't count calories or even know how many calories are in each food item, yet they never appear to put on weight or have any issues with weight.

It was when I finally worked out how these people managed to enjoy eating and maintain their healthy weight, that I finally understood the answer to real and permanent weight loss while still enjoying eating. The key point about all of the naturally healthy-weight people I observed is that they don't work hard at weight management - on the contrary!

When I thought back to the time in my life when I was at *my* healthy-weight, I didn't work hard either. It was only when I fell into the *bad eating habits* and moved away from the good natural eating habits I had been conditioned to do as a child and followed until I was in my mid-twenties, that I started to become gradually overweight. And every time I went on a diet, I always became more over weight.

Maybe you are like me and can look back at a time when you were at your naturally healthy-weight and didn't worry about counting calories, etc.

I had a good look at myself and analysed *why* I had moved up from being at my naturally healthy-weight and fit up to my mid-twenties, to becoming an increasingly overweight couch potato. I decided that I wanted to be like the naturally healthy-weight people I had been thinking about, and find out how they were able to live in the same world I do, surrounded with the same tempting food, and not put on the weight in the way that I had done over the years.

I explore this in the next chapter.

Chapter 4

Why do some people 'naturally' never put on weight?

I discovered the answer to this question and it became the key to my success in losing weight and sustaining the weight loss.

Before I address this question I am going to address some come common myths:

Myth buster: *'I am naturally big so there is no point trying to lose weight'.*

It is true that people come in all shapes and sizes and some people can be bigger than others; however, no one should be *'overweight'*. Someone is overweight when they are heavier than their individual ideal weight for their height and build.

Please do not use the old 'I am naturally big and meant to be this size'. It is vital for the sake of your health to work out the ideal healthy weight for your natural build. Remember, we are looking at how you can achieve the *ideal healthy-weight that is appropriate for you!*

Myth buster: *'My metabolism is naturally slow, unlike these naturally healthy-weight people who are lucky enough to have been born with a naturally fast metabolism'*

This is partly true as we do differ in our metabolism; however, our metabolism can be changed and influenced by how we eat. It is a nice excuse to blame it for our lack of weight loss. I am sorry to tell you that you cannot blame your metabolism. Please read the section on 'Metabolism' for a more detailed analysis.

Myth buster: *'I have cut down on my food and I really don't eat that much, yet I never lose any weight'.*

This used to be one of my favourite cop-outs. I am sorry to have to tell you that if you are overweight, just like I was, it is because you are eating too much and not eating in the way you have been created and designed to eat. To achieve and maintain our ideal healthy-weight, we must follow Nature's way by providing the proper nutrients which will 'fuel' our body in the most efficient and appropriate way. I used to kid myself by believing this myth!

Your failure to lose weight is the result of a number of factors. Perhaps you are trying to *'stick to a diet'* (remember, diets don't work), or you may be a *'secret eater'* or *'emotional eater'*. Please read the relevant sections of this book under these headings for a more detailed analysis of these topics.

Myth buster: '*As we get older we naturally put on weight and it is natural to get bigger and fatter'; therefore, there is no point trying to lose weight – I am now meant to be this weight at my age'.*

This is only partly true – we may get slightly heavier, but we are not meant to become overweight. We become overweight because we *let* ourselves become overweight. I know what I am talking about because I gradually allowed myself to develop from a slim fit person into an overweight couch potato by convincing myself that this particular myth was true. I now know better.

It is true that many people do become increasingly overweight as they age, but this is not inevitable. As we age we usually reduce our activity and don't burn as many calories because we don't need as much 'fuel'. Unfortunately, we don't adjust the amount of food that we consume and this will result in a surplus of calories. The body can only do one thing with the unused surplus of calories – turn them into fat and store them.

Now back to the naturally healthy-weight person.

As I stated in the previous chapter, after carefully studying the eating habits of naturally healthy-weight people in my circle of family and friends, and thinking carefully back to the time when I didn't have a weight problem, I realised a very simple and vitally important truth. I realised that these people actually are not overweight because they follow a few very basic eating habits or patterns. I realised that *I actually used these eating habits in the past without knowing it.*

It was when I moved away from these eating habits that I started to become fat and unfit.

What are these eating habits required to enable you to achieve your natural healthy-weight, and maintain it the natural way?

I realised after watching these naturally healthy-weight people that they sub-consciously follow certain fundamental principles. Also, thinking back to days before I put on weight, I realised that I also followed these principles without thinking about it:

- Only eat when actually genuinely hungry (in response to the hunger hormone *Ghrelin* in your *stomach*, not your imagination).
- Eat your food slowly.
- Stop eating when you feel full (your body releases the hormone *Leptin* to let you know when it has had enough food.

I realised that I had heard these principles all of my childhood and used to follow these rules naturally without thinking. I can think back to meal times when I was a child and being told the following eating guidelines by my wise parents: *'eat slowly and chew your food'; 'don't confuse greed with need'; 'listen to your tummy and not your head'; 'eat when your stomach tells you that you are hungry'* and *'stop and don't eat any more food than your tummy tells you it needs it.'*

This wisdom was freely offered and drummed into me by my parents and other wise adults; however, as is the complacency of youth, I never really appreciated that they we instilling into me key principles, based on an instinctive understanding of the natural way we have been created to eat.

I was amazed to think back and realise that this wisdom was being freely offered without thinking by my parents and others of influence during my childhood. I followed this wisdom right up until my mid-twenties. At this point; I stopped following this 'natural' way of eating and stared to fall into the bad eating habits that led to my becoming overweight. I then started to fall into the diet trap, and became even heavier after each failed diet attempt

Thankfully, I have re-discovered this 'natural' way and I have lost all of the extra weight I gained (four and a half stone/sixty three pounds). I am writing this book to help you escape the diet trap and lose weight the natural way by following these simple principles and become like the naturally healthy-weight person you live and work with, or maybe used to be at some point in the past.

All the naturally healthy-weight people I observed also followed these rules without thinking.

What does science have to say about weight-gain?

There obviously must be a scientific explanation for why some people are (and I used to be) naturally healthy-weight.

I came to the conclusion that it was important to understand the *science* and *psychology* behind why these people don't struggle with weight-gain – seemingly without effort, diets, calorie-counting, etc. Therefore, it was important to try to understand the science of *how* the body processes the food we eat, and the *psychology* behind *why* people struggle with weight.

I concluded that if I could understand and 'tune in' to the scientific and natural way we are designed to eat in the most efficient way, I would have found the best way to lose weight and maintain the best health-weight for me. You can't beat Nature!

I concentrated my reading on science and medical text books and articles, and read about anatomy & physiology, neuro-science, and psychology, etc., explaining the scientific technicalities of how the body is naturally designed to eat and process food, and how our attitude of mind can affect our eating.

The result of this personal study led me to totally change my approach to weight loss.

<u>Don't just take my word for it</u>

I was quite sure that I had discovered the best way to lose weight; however, I also wanted to be more confident that I was on the right track.

I had already read and rejected many of the various 'diet' books and programmes available. My rejection of these was based on my failed attempts to lose weight by following these programmes.

My next strategy was to start reading and studying what others had to say on the subject of losing weight *without* going on a 'diet'.

I was both intrigued and encouraged by the fact that so many of these books and articles had actually come more or less to the same conclusion that I had, albeit in different words. We were all saying basically the same thing. The only way to lose weight in a real and lasting way was to adopt the natural way our bodies had been designed to eat, and to re-educate our eating habits by adapting a few simple principles. Current TV ads and healthy eating campaigns from good organisations also say the same thing!

This is consistent with the old sayings 'The truth in Nature is consistent' and 'All truth is God's truth'.

The result of all of the aforementioned thought, observation and personal research was to highlight to me that the natural, most effective way to lose weight in a real and effective way, can be summed up in an approach which I think is as easy as'1, 2, 3.'

Chapter 5
Weight loss is as easy as *'1, 2, 3'*

Time for an illustration:

Think about that lovely car you have just paid for with your hard-earned cash (or by loan or credit agreement). How do you make sure that you keep the car going in the best and most reliable way possible? Simple answer, you will follow the manufacturer's instructions carefully and make sure that you use the correct fuel, maintain the correct oil level and tyre pressure, add the right type and amount of coolant and brake fluid, etc. In other words, you will maintain it the way is designed to be maintained.

What happens if you move away from maintaining it the way has been designed to be maintained? Simple answer, it will develop faults and break down. Most people would not dream of being as careless about maintaining their car as they are about maintaining their body.

In the same way, we need to look after the fantastic 'machine' that is our body by making sure we maintain it in a way that is consistent with how it has been designed to function, if we want to keep it going in a healthy and efficient way. If we put the wrong components into our car then we know that it will not function efficiently and eventually break down.

Question: How do we make sure that we are maintaining the 'machine' that is our body in the most efficient way that is consistent with how we have been created and with the maintenance rules in the 'manufacturer's handbook' (the laws of Nature)?

Answer: The answer is simple and logical – we look at how we have been created to eat and follow the most efficient eating habits determined and demanded by the laws of Nature, by doing so, we will find that eating to achieve and maintain a healthy weight will become natural part of our everyday life.

Question: Does this mean that we need to become a scientist and study how Nature affects our body, if we are to make sure we are following eating patterns which are consistent with how we have been designed to eat and nourish our bodies?

Answer: Absolutely not! Nature is brilliant at making the things we need to know easily understood – if we are prepared to 'listen' to Nature and follow the key natural rules required for survival and quality of life. It is when we humans decide that we know better than Nature and formulate our own way of doing things (like diet programmes) that things go wrong. We must not over complicate things as Nature knows best.

Question: What are the fantastically simple 'rules of Nature' that we can follow, if we want to make sure that we are eating and achieving a healthy weight in a way that is consistent with how we have been created (as consistent with the rules of Nature)?

Answer: There are different ways of summarising these rules, and they all say more or less the same thing, albeit with different wording; however, my summary of the process I followed to lose weight is as simple as '1, 2, 3'. I call it the '*Three Point Plan*'.

The plan is:

1. Eat only when you are genuinely hungry - in your stomach, not your imagination (or 'tummy hungry' to use the old well-known phrase).

Learn to 'listen' to your body when it releases the hunger hormone (Ghrelin) to let you know it is time to eat and're-fuel' your body with food.

2. Eat slowly.

Slow down, chew your food slowly and do not scoff the food down – as your may have been told when you were a child.

3. Stop eating when you feel that your stomach feels full.

Learn to 'listen' to your body when it naturally sends the chemical (Leptin) to let you know your stomach it is full.

Please note that I have not mentioned anything about what food that you can and can't eat as this is not a diet and no food has been banned.

It is <u>not</u> about cutting out this food or that food – it is about re-educating or changing your eating habits and listening to when your body tells you that it is time to eat.

Yes, it is that easy and straightforward.

You do not need to punish yourself or stick to some hard diet programme. As already stated, these diet programmes do not work in the long term. You may have some weight loss; but, the weight will return.

Willpower does not work. Weight loss is about making eating correctly part of the normal routine of your everyday life. You need to re-educate your eating habits, not starve or deprive yourself.

The only way to lose weight and get fit on a real and lasting way is to make the new eating habit part of your everyday life.

Remember, overeating is a *habit* - you have learned how to overeat.

To achieve lasting weight loss you must replace the bad eating habits that you have developed over a long period of time. This is easier than you think – certainly easier than following some fad diet.

To re-emphasise what I have said before, I lost four and a half stone (sixty three pounds) following this method and have kept the weight off.

Remember, this book is not another diet programme, rather it is a guide into a journey for you to follow to find the natural way for you to lose weight - the way your body was designed to do so.

It is only when you follow the natural way – the way your body was designed to operate, that you will actuality achieve weigh loss that is real and permanent.

You need to develop and establish the ***process*** of ***how*** you ***should*** eat. Believe me, this is much easier than trying to force yourself to 'stick' to a diet which won't work in the long term.

Once you have mastered the natural *process* of ***how*** you should eat, we can then look in more detail at ***what*** foods we should eat.

This is turning on its head the key approach of 'going on a diet', which states that you must constantly worry and monitor 'what' you eat, and using willpower. This is wrong and doomed to failure because you are going against how you have been created and naturally & genetically programmed – you are fighting Nature.

You are doing the same as King Canute who according legend sat on his throne at the sea shore and tried to order the tide not to come on to the beach.

Trying to lose weight on a permanent basis by going on a diet is just as much of a futile waste of time. *You cannot beat Nature!*

Medical conditions:

'I have a medical condition which causes weight gain. Is there any point in me following the Three Point Plan?'

Yes, definitely! Some medical conditions cause weight gain as either a symptom or side effect of medication. This plan can help you achieve the healthiest weight possible for ***you*** within the context of your condition.

Chapter 6

Diet Warning

Do not make it too complicated for yourself!

I have discovered an interesting reaction when people ask me how I managed to lose the weight and keep it off for so long.

When I tell them they are almost disappointed because I did not follow some drastic diet programme involving strong willpower, sacrifice, harsh cutting out of all sorts of nice foods, etc.

It seems that we have become conditioned into believing that we must punish ourselves with hard self-sacrificing diets if we are going to lose weight.

I know because I used to be caught in this trap until I realised that punishing myself with strict diets and using willpower just didn't work.

Please do not fall into this trap – *learn from my mistakes*, and please learn from how I eventually lost weight permanently.

Losing weight and becoming fit & healthy in a real, long-lasting and natural way can be achieved by following the approach outlined in this book. I am not quoting theory – I am quoting my experience!

I wasted so much time and energy punishing myself on 'diets' which only brought about short term results and more weight gain. Remember, diets do not work for the majority of people.

Chapter 7

The benefits of losing weight

This may appear to be so obvious that it is not worth writing about; however, I found that thinking about these things often helped me to stay focused on all that I needed to do when I was in the early stages of my weight loss journey.

When I was overweight I didn't fully appreciate the negative impact my obesity had on my physical, mental and emotional health and well-being. I used to say that I was happy enough and had come to terms with being overweight.

I realise now that I was kidding myself. The truth is obvious to me now when I look back – I was not happy about my weight.

You are reading this book because deep down you too are not happy about your weight. Perhaps you are very well aware of how unhappy you are, or perhaps like me, you are kidding yourself and in denial!

I also suffered from physical and health problems when I was overweight. I had high blood pressure, high cholesterol and suffered from a chronic lack of energy.

Some of the many benefits of weight loss and improved fitness are:

- More energy and better general health.
- Better immune system.
- Better moods and more self-confidence.

Chapter 8

Metabolism

Metabolism is a very commonly used word by people who are overweight. I am very well aware of this because I used this term a lot.

'It is because of my metabolism that I am overweight' is the cry of many an overweight person. It is a very good cop-out and one that I used to justify my growing midriff as I moved from being a naturally healthy-weight to an overweight couch potato.

Can we really say that our weight problem is because of our metabolism?

Actually, the answer is no.

In reality, we can make our metabolism 'go more slowly' because of our bad eating habits. On the other hand, the metabolism can also be 'speeded up' when we re-educate our bad eating habits to the natural habits we have been looking at in this book.

Here is a straightforward layman's explanation of metabolism for those of you, who like me, are not scientists.

The simplest definition that I can give regarding metabolism is that it is the speed at which our body creates the energy needed to do all the things that keeps us alive and healthy. This energy is created by the body taking the food we eat and turning it into energy. This energy will be used for every living process in our body from hair growth to the regulation of our heart rate.

Significantly, from the point of view of this book about weight loss, our metabolism will regulate the process and speed at which the body will burn off fat and calories every day.

The faster your metabolism, the faster and more efficiently your body will burn off the fat. Conversely, the slower your metabolic rate, the more slowly and less efficiently your body will burn off fat.

This means that somebody who is overweight and unfit will usually burn calories and fat at a much slower rate than someone who is at a naturally healthy-weight for them as an individual. This is why so many overweight people blame the fact that they are overweight on the idea that they have a naturally slow metabolism.

When they think about their weight and the fact that they are not getting lighter, they will cry *'it is not my fault that I am overweight! I have been dealt a bad hand by Nature, which has genetically given me a slow metabolism'.*

As we have established, it is true that people who are overweight usually do have a slower metabolism resulting in calories and fat being burned a slower rate; however, let's ask the key question from the point of view of weight loss – *'is this the chicken or the egg?'*

Question: Are we overweight because of a slow metabolism, or is our metabolism slow because we are overweight?

The answer to this is very significant for those of us who long to lose weight.

If we are born genetically programmed to have a slow metabolism which leads to us inevitably becoming overweight, then this is bad news as we 'cannot help' being overweight because of our metabolism.

On the other hand, if our metabolism slows down because we *become* overweight, then this is good news because it means that we are not doomed by genetics to be overweight as the result of the slow metabolism. It also means that we cannot use 'slow metabolism' as an excuse for being overweight.

So, which is it?

Are some people born with a slow metabolism that condemns them to be overweight? Or do they slow down their own metabolism by overeating and eating the wrong foods in the wrong way?

Thankfully, the great news is that the second statement is true, and we can change our metabolism by changing how we eat and treat our body in our everyday life.

This assertion is based upon current credible and authoritative research, which has demonstrated that our metabolism is not set at a certain level and can be changed – either in a negative or positive way!

We know now that we can change our metabolism in an unhelpful way by 'slowing it down'.

How exactly do we do this?

There appears to be three main ways that are relevant to our discussion about weight loss:

- Eating too much of the wrong food.
- Not enough activity.
- Going 'on a diet' in an attempt to lose weight.

Yes, I will emphasise the third point again:

Going 'on a diet' in an attempt to lose weight can actually cause your metabolism to slow down, which will contribute to your weight gain!

This is because a slower metabolism is less efficient at burning fat and calories. Therefore, you will not be able to lose weight in a real and lasting way!

Therefore, we have another clear reason that proves why <u>diets do not work</u>!

The obvious question now is: how do we reverse the 'slow metabolism' that we have created by our bad eating habits and lack of appropriate activity levels?

The answer is actually very straightforward:

- Re-educate your eating habits by following the *'Three Point Plan'* outlined in this book.
- Increase your physical activity.

What do I mean by increase physical activity? I mean exactly what I say – you need to engage in some sort of physical activity that results in the speed of your heart beat increasing and your lungs expanding because you need to breathe more deeply.

You are now probably thinking about the dreaded 'e' word – exercise!

Please don't panic when you think of this word. I am going to look briefly at the difference between *exercise* and *exercise programmes*.

You are already doing *exercise* everyday as it is *movement* of any kind and includes, walking, using a vacuum cleaner, dusting, cooking, loading the washing machine, hanging out the washing, looking after young children, etc. I call this *'Level 'A' activity'* and will be the *foundation of your fitnes*s!

You can add to your current level of 'exercise' by putting more effort into your daily activities, thus causing your heart and breathing rate to increase.

Exercise programmes are the activities you do in *addition* the 'exercise' (normal movement and activities of daily life – 'Level A') you do already, and include things such as running, swimming, going to the gym, etc. I call this '*Level B'* activity.

I will explore these concepts in more depth in the specific chapter *Exercise*.

The key thing to remember about this chapter is:

- Your metabolism is 'slowed down' because of your bad eating and lifestyle habits.
- Your metabolism is not fixed and can be change and 'speeded up' by re-educating your eating and lifestyle habits, including 'moving more'!
- Because your metabolism can be 'slowed down' and 'speeded up' by either your good or bad eating and life style habits, *you cannot use metabolism as an excuse for the fact that you are overweight!*

Chapter 9

Counting calories can make you fat

This statement may come as a shock as you may be thinking, as I used to, that counting calories is the very thing that you should be doing in order to lose weight.

We have been conditioned into thinking that calorie counting is the most fundamentally important aspect of weight loss and the foundation of most diet programmes.

This is in fact one of the many reasons why diets do not work. It is a false foundation upon which diets are built.

Am I saying that calories are not important? Of course not; however, we must put calories into the appropriate context and use our knowledge about calories in the correct way.

We need to be *aware* of calories, but strict counting them will not work. Remember, diets do not work and this is not a diet programme!

One of the lessons I learned from my failed diet attempts is that I really could not sustain the ongoing detailed calorie counting, which was the requirement of the diets I was trying to follow.

It became a real chore trying to work out how many calories there were in every item of food I wanted to eat. I got fed up with the maths of trying to work out what I could eat in order to maintain a healthy weight.

This conscious food restriction based on the maths of calorie counting was not working for me. I did lose some weight; however, as the calorie counting is unsustainable in the long run, I always ended up getting fatter. I also always found it a miserable experience, which is another reason why calorie counting is unsustainable – it was having a negative psychological effect.

Counting calories is also not an accurate way of measuring the effect your overall food intake will have on your weight. This is important to understand as sometimes we can justify to ourselves the eating of a certain food because it has 'so many calories' contained in it and this will keep us within our 2000 calorie daily limit (or whatever the individual limit has been set).

Let us think about this objectively.

A 330ml can of a popular cola-type drink contains approximately 140 calories. Contrast this with a food type that contains a similar amount of calories - a Chicken breast that has been cooked in the most health conscious way (without the skin and grilled).

Can you really say that consuming 140 calories by drinking a can of the popular cola-type drink has the same impact on your weight management as eating a healthy grilled skinless chicken breast?

Of course not, as the cola-type drink will contain a lot of other ingredients which are the enemy of weight loss – especially the high amount of *sugar!*

In contrast, when you eat the 140 or so calories in the grilled skinless chicken breast, you are not only avoiding the substances that are bad for your waistline such as large amounts of sugar; you are also putting in things such as protein which is good for the health of your body.

Therefore, while you should be *aware* of calories, there are far more things to think about than just the *amount* of calories. If we don't think about these other factors and eat food based just on calorie counting, we run the danger that we underestimate and miscalculate the overall effect that some of the foods we eat can have on our weight management.

Therefore, depending on your approach, *counting calories can make you fat*

Chapter 10

The baby, the squirrel, the mice & cheesecake, the cat & the cream and the bear and honey

I enjoy watching documentaries about Nature and science. It is always great to learn something new about the marvellous world in which we live. We cannot do better for our full potential well-being than look at the laws of Nature and apply the key principles to our life.

I have repeatedly been saying that diets do not work and we must tune into how we have been created to eat and programmed by natural laws to feed our body, if it is going to function in the most effective way possible.

I will illustrate what I mean by sharing some of the observations I made and conclusions I arrived at by watching documentaries on the following topics: The development of a baby, the squirrel preparing for winter, a scientific experiment with mice and cheesecake and the habits of cats and bears.

The Baby

Think about a newborn baby – when it is hungry, it will cry for food. When he or she has had their fill of their mother's milk – they will stop taking the milk. Nature has provided babies with a natural 'off switch' when it comes to how much food they need to take in.

Remarkably, as the baby grows and develops in size, he or she will still only take in the amount of milk they need as appropriate to their nutritional needs.

As the baby continues to grow, he or she will eventually naturally come off milk and move on to solids.

A baby has an inbuilt system of food modification and intake regulation. It will only eat what it needs, and this is the key to real weight loss and weight management.

We become overweight when we allow ourselves ignore the natural signals from our body to eat when we are truly hungry in our stomach ('tummy hungry') and to stop when we have taken all the nourishment we need and feel sufficiently full.

We adults still have this natural inbuilt system of food modification and intake regulation. Why then do we overeat and become overweight? The answer is simple. We have allowed ourselves to be conditioned by the culture and society we live in into eating in a way that we were not genetically programmed to do.

Remember, it is when we stop listening to our body and the natural signals regarding when we should eat and when we should stop eating that we become overweight. The secret to weight loss is not diets – it is re-learning to listen to how we are naturally meant to eat – just like the baby.

The squirrel

It goes without saying that there is much more to Nature and the natural world than the human race.

We humans can learn so much from looking at the whole of Nature and think about the lessons we can learn from the other animal species who share this planet with us.

We will now look at a couple of examples from the animal kingdom which illustrate and are consistent with the key points of this natural weight-loss programme.

Take the squirrel for example. I watched a fascinating documentary about a squirrel preparing for winter.

The documentary highlighted that even in a situation where there is an abundance of nuts, the squirrel will eat so much and store the rest.

The key fact from our point of view is the squirrel has a natural 'off switch' with regards to eating enough for its needs.

We too have an 'off switch'; unfortunately, through bad eating habits established as a result of cultural conditioning, we have lost the art of paying attention to this 'off switch'. One of the key secrets in losing weight and keeping it off permanently and naturally is to learn how to tune into this 'off switch'.

Mice and the cheesecake.

I watched a fascinating science documentary about experiments on mice and their reaction to cheesecake, and was struck by how relevant it was to my personal study and research into the most effective way to permanently lose weight.

Unfortunately I can't remember the details of where, when or by whom the experiments were carried out; however, I do remember the gist of the experiment, and how the results reinforces the suggestion that nature has equipped us with an 'off switch' to regulate how we are naturally designed to eat, and how we can be conditioned into not 'listening' to this natural 'off switch'.

The experiments on mice

The purpose of the experiments was to investigate if there was a link between the type of food we eat and why we eat it. In other words, can the actual structure and content of the food actually change the way we eat it and the amount we eat?

The experiments were organised along these lines:

The First Experiment:

The mice were fed a total diet consisting only of sugar, and significantly, they could eat as much as they wanted – there were no restrictions.

The result of this total sugar diet was quite startling. Despite the fact they only had access to a sugar-based diet, and could eat as much as they wanted, *they did not put on any weight.*

The mice would eat a certain amount and then stop. It appears that they had this natural 'off switch'. The mice seemed to know and to obey the signal from their bodies to stop eating.

The Second Experiment:

This experiment was conducted along the same lines as the first. However, this time the mice were fed a diet consisting only of *fat*.

Again, as in the first experiment with the sugar, they could eat as much as they wanted – there were no restrictions.

Remarkably, the result of this total-fat diet was as startling and significant as the sugar experiment. Again, despite the fact that they only had access to a fat-based diet, and could eat as much as they wanted, *they did not put on any weight.*

The mice would eat a certain amount of the fat diet and then stop. It appears that, as with the sugar diet, they had a natural 'off switch' that is given by Nature. The mice seemed to know and to obey the signal from their bodies to stop eating.

The third experiment:

The mice were fed a mixture of fat and sugar. This was fed to them in the form of cheesecake.

The results of this experiment were truly remarkable. In complete contrast to the results of the previous two experiments, the mice actually put on a great deal of weight. In fact, they became morbidly obese and very sedentary and slept a lot.

The results of this experiment demonstrated that it was clear that when the mice followed the diet where the fat and sugar was combined in equal amounts, there was no 'off switch' as there had been with either fat or sugar only. The mice just loved this combination and did not stop eating.

Question: Why did the mice stop obeying the natural signals from their bodies when they ate this combination of fat and sugar?

Answer: this combination of fat and sugar is *not found in nature*!

Question: Why is this significant?

Answer: this combination of fat and sugar, which is not found in nature, is human-created or 'processed food'. The mice had been 'conditioned' by this to ignore their natural 'off switch', and had put on weight as a result.

Summary of the mice and cheesecake experiment result:

Experiment	Food type eaten exclusively by the mice	Effect on weight	Conclusion
1	Sugar	No weight gain	There appeared to be a natural *'off switch'* which naturally stopped them from eating too much.
2	Fat	No weight gain	There appeared to be a natural *'off switch'* which naturally stopped them from eating too much.

3	Fat & Sugar combined (50/50)	Massive weight gain	The combination of sugar & fat (processed food) appeared to cause the mice to 'ignore' the natural 'off switch'. This type of processed food does not exist in nature.

Why is this relevant to our study of weight loss management?

To put this into context, we must understand that we have two generically programmed appetite pathways which run parallel with and complement each other. I will be looking at these in more detail later; however, I give a brief introduction now in order for this illustration of the mice experiment to make sense.

What are these two complementary genetically programmed appetite pathways?

The *Homeostatic* eating appetite pathway: recognises and triggers eating food as fuel to keep our body alive.

The *Hedonic* eating and appetite pathway: recognises that we must also eat for pleasure and enjoyment of food.

Yes, that is correct – we have been created and genetically programmed to actually *enjoy* the food we eat. It is hot-wired into our DNA that eating should be enjoyable. This runs parallel to the obvious fact that we need to eat food to fuel our body and keep it alive.

This is a fact of Nature and it should be celebrated! As long as we keep these two genetically programmed appetite pathways *balanced correctly.*

If we move away from the correct balance between eating to live and eating for pleasure, we are creating problems for ourselves and creating the weight-management problems which contribute to our 'battle of the bulge' and expanding waistline.

The eating for *pleasure* (Hedonic) is the 'servant' to the eating to *stay alive* (Homeostatic), and will be a source of our weight-management difficulties if make it the master and not the servant.

More about these appetite pathways later – now, back to the mice and the cheesecake!

When the mice ate the combination of fat and sugar (the cheesecake), the fat and sugar mixture appeared to trigger the part of the brain which decides that we 'like eating food' (Hedonic system) as opposed to the part of the brain that tells us to 'eat to live' (Homeostatic system).

In other words, they stopped obeying the genetically programmed chemical signals which told them that they had eaten enough food to stay alive, and were inadvertently letting the 'eating for pleasure' aspect take over.

The cat and the cream

Let's look at another example from another informative documentary about Nature to illustrate this further.

I watched a fascinating documentary about one of our most popular pets – the cat.

Cats are amazing creatures. They are self-reliant, athletic and agile - just think about their ability to jump, climb and balance. It has been said that we don't own our pet cat; rather, the cat chooses to honour us with the presence of its company, and gives us the privilege of looking after it.

Our pet cat will stay with us as long as we feed and water it in a home that provides it with comfort and warmth.

Cats will eat the food that we give it; however; the 'negative' side of the cat's nature from our point of view, is that it will also catch and kill other creatures. This does create a dislike of cats among some people.

The cat will prefer to have its 'owner' open a tin and place meat into a dish and set it down in front of it. The owner is the person to whom it has decided to give the honour of looking after it.

It is much easier for the cat to torture the 'owner' for food by constantly meowing until the point of overload, and to walk around the feet until the fear of the real threat of tripping over the cat brings the owner to breaking point and sets the food down.

This saves the cat from the bother of hunting and catching its own dinner. However, the cat will follow its instinct to catch other creatures. If the cat is not hungry, it will play with the poor creature it has caught. If the cat is hungry and needs food, it will eat the unfortunate prey. It will do this to satisfy its natural need to eat to live (Homeostatic appetite pathway).

A cat does not only eat to live. If you put down some cream, it will also eagerly follow its natural instinct to take the eating-for-pleasure (Hedonic) appetite pathway.

The bear and the honey

One more illustration from the lessons I have learned from the world of Nature and science documentaries - the bear and the honey!

The documentary was about life in a forest somewhere in North America. Sorry, but once again I can't remember the exact details.

The programme turned its focus to a hollowed-out tree which had become home to a colony of honeybees. A large bear emerged from the depths of the forest and stood watching this tree beehive. The bear was interested in one thing – the *honey*! It moved in and put its large paw into the hive and pulled out a large piece of honey.

The bees obviously followed their natural instinct to defend the hive and attacked and stung the bear.

However, the bear endured the stings for as long as it could and scooped as much honey as possible before the unrelenting multiple stings of the bees became too much to endure any longer.

Question: Why did the bear put itself into such a painful situation?

Answer: Because of the natural desire to eat for pleasure (Hedonic appetite pathway). The bear followed its natural desire to eat and enjoy Nature's sweet gift – *honey!*

What are the lessons relevant to weight management we can learn from these documentaries?

- We have been created with two parallel appetite pathways. Homeostatic (eating to keep our body alive) and Hedonic (eating for pleasure and enjoyment of food).

- We must become 'tuned in' to these facts, and establish good natural eating habits, which are consistent with the natural appetite instincts we have been born with.

- Processed food is not found in nature and thus is a real enemy to healthy weight management.

Does this mean that we can't eat processed food such as cheesecake?

No, however, we must re-educate our eating habits and follow the natural parallel appetite pathways to make sure that we don't eat too much – and in particular, too much of the *wrong* type of food.

Chapter 11

Homeostatic and Hedonic appetite pathways.

In the previous chapter, we thought about the two parallel appetite pathways we have been naturally equipped with – the Homeostatic (eating to live) and Hedonic (eating for pleasure).

Let's look at these in a little more detail, as it is essential to understand the significance of these appetite pathways, if we are going to fully develop the new and appropriate eating habits we need to manage our weight.

I am sure that you have watched on TV those documentaries where some survival expert is on a remote island or jungle somewhere far away from civilisation.

Food will obviously be difficult to come by in this remote place – no shops to nip into and do the weekly shopping. The person needs to eat and get the right nutrients to live; however, where is he or she going to get the nutrition?

In order to answer this, the survival expert will pick up some strange looking insect and tell us about all of the nutrition we can get if we eat that odd looking little creature. He or she will then eat it and tell us that the taste of the insect is disgusting, but it will keep us alive.

Just think for a moment about how joyless life would be if eating only involved eating flavourless but healthy food items to stay alive, without any regard to taste and enjoyment! Eating the insect would be consistent with the Homeostatic, eating-to-live appetite pathway, but it would be awful to live this way!

Fortunately, we do not just eat to live. We have also been given the Hedonic pathway so that we *enjoy* eating our food as well as eating the things that keep us alive.

Why do you think we find things in Nature such as *honey*! The sole purpose of honey is to provide us a natural food stuff that we can eat purely for enjoyment.

We should not feel guilty about enjoying our food. Neither should we feel guilty about eating treats.

However, the problem arises when we place too much emphasis on the Hedonic (pleasure eating) and it grows out of proportion.

The Hedonic (pleasure) appetite should be the servant, not the master. If we let it become the master, the result will be an ever expanding waistline!

Summary

Homeostatic eating/hunger: recognises and triggers eating food as fuel/eat to live.

Hedonic eating/hunger: triggers eating food for pleasure, enjoyment and reward.

Both are essential for humans, however, both must be in correct balance for healthy eating.

Chapter 12

Why do we eat? What is hunger?

1. Why do we eat?

The answer is surely obvious! You are probably thinking 'we eat to live' and 'we eat because we are hungry'.

You are partly right – we *should* eat because we are hungry and because we need to eat to live; however, most of us who are or have been overweight actually overeat because we don't just stick to eating the way we have been genetically programmed to do (i.e. in order to live and because we are hungry).

No, we eat, or perhaps I should say, we *overeat* for a number of different reasons.

Some of these are:

- Bad habit.
- Emotional reasons (comfort eating).
- Eating because we like it! Remember 'the experiment on mice' and their love of the combination of fat and sugar?

2. What is hunger?

Again, this at first sight may appear to be a silly question with an obvious answer. But in fact, once you understand the significance of the answer to this question, you will be well on your way to achieving the new eating habits that will help you achieve the weight loss that you are looking and longing for.

We must understand the following key points:

- There is a difference between genuine *hunger in the stomach* (tummy hunger) and *hunger in the imagination* (head hunger).
- We have two appetite pathways that regulate our food intake (Homeostatic and Hedonic).
- We are conditioned (influenced and have our thoughts and habits set) by our culture, society and upbringing.

If we are overweight, we are following the bad habits taught to and *negatively* conditioned into us. If we are the correct and healthy weight, then we have been *positively* conditioned to eat the genetically natural way.

I am delighted to be able to tell you that if we have adopted negative eating patterns, we can be re-educated into finding positive ones.

Now, let's get back to the question: 'What is hunger?'

My answer to this question changed completely when I decided to research into how to lose weight the natural way.

One of the major lessons I learned from my personal research is that our understanding and interpretation of hunger will actually have a direct impact on our weight. Remember, hunger is a natural process and it is a marvellous thing. Your body is fantastic at keeping you alive.

Hunger is also a *complicated* process. Here is how it works:

Different chemicals are released by the body to act upon the signal from the brain that our bodies are in need of fuel. The main chemical is *Ghrelin.*

Different chemicals are also released to tell us when we have had enough food to fuel our bodies – a type of 'off switch'. The main chemical is *Leptin.*

Ghrelin	Tells us that our body needs to eat to provide fuel for our body
Leptin	Tells us when we have had enough food (fuel)

When we are born we naturally tune in to and 'listen' these signals to start eating when we need to, and to stop when we are full.

One of the reasons I became overweight was I had lost the ability to tell the difference between *genuine hunger in the stomach* (tummy hunger)' and *hunger in the imagination* (head hunger).

Genuine hunger in the stomach (tummy hunger): This is the 'natural' hunger when the hunger hormone (Ghrelin) is released into our body to tell us that we need food.

Hunger in the imagination (head hunger). This is the 'unnatural' or 'bad habit' hunger that makes us wrongly think that we need to take food, or certain types of food. We are conditioned into head hunger through bad habit, cultural pressure, etc.

When we can tell the *difference* between *genuine* and *imagined* hunger, we will be able to lose weight the natural way and stay at a healthy weight.

What happens when you are naturally hungry tummy hungry?

Food is the fuel that keeps the body moving and living. Think about your car for a moment. Petrol is the thing that keeps your car moving. When the petrol tank is running low in fuel, a sensor in the petrol tank sends a signal via the electric system of the car to the warning light on the dashboard. This tells you that the car needs more fuel to keep moving. A similar thing happens in your body.

When the body detects that it is running low in fuel it will send a signal to the brain by means of a chemical released by the stomach and pancreas – this chemical is called *Ghrelin.*

Ghrelin is the hunger hormone.

Hunger comes on slowly and gradually - a little bit at a time. It will start as a twinge or mild sensation in your stomach region. This is the beginning of your body realising that it is getting low on fuel and releasing the hunger hormone. This sensation will gradually grow and build in intensity until your stomach starts to 'growl' and will eventually feel pain.

It is essential to be able to recognise this 'natural' hunger signal and learn to change our faulty eating habits if we want to lose weight.

In other words, natural hunger is a *physical* process that lets your mind know that more fuel is needed.

There is a parallel between this, and the natural process of needing to use the toilet to eliminate waste when our bowels need to move.

In fact, they are the beginning (hunger signal to take in fuel) and end (eliminate the waste product) of the same refuelling process.

When we need to go to the toilet, we are alerted by means of a sensation in our body as it sends us a signal. This signal will only be a slight sensation at the beginning. Eventually, it will become stronger and stronger, until it becomes so strong that we can no longer ignore it and must act!

In the same way, the feeling of genuine hunger in the stomach (tummy hunger) begins with a slight sensation in the tummy area. Eventually, the signal that we are hungry and need food to refuel our body will grow until it becomes too strong for us to ignore.

Parallel	
Hunger	Physical instinct and sensation that will build gradually.
Needing the toilet	Physical instinct and sensation that will build gradually

Remember the lesson from the baby in an earlier chapter?

Babies are obviously not born with the ability to understand and communicate their needs. They are dependent on what is technically referred to as the 'primitive reflexes'.

When they are hungry a chemical signal (Ghrelin) is sent from the tummy to the brain informing it that it needs more fuel. The baby will then instinctively communicate its need for fuel by means of the only tool for communication it has at this stage – it will cry.

Interestingly, usually the baby will suckle slowly and will *stop* when it is satisfied that it has received sufficient fuel. This happens because the baby will instinctively react to the natural chemical (*Leptin*) released to inform the brain that it has had enough, thus following the natural eating process present from birth.

This basic hunger pattern is the blueprint for how we should eat to function as we have been created. The problem arises when we grow up and fall into bad eating habits.

Hunger in the imagination (head hunger).

This is the biggest threat to our waistline!

True hunger is in the *stomach*; however, weight gain happens when we have become used to thinking about hunger in our *head*.

Chapter 13

Secret eaters, Emotional Eaters, Habit Eaters

Are you a secret eater? I was.

What do I mean by 'secret eater'?

I used to convince myself that I did not eat all that much; however, I could not understand why my 'diets' and 'cutting out' did not achieve any weight loss – the opposite in fact – I always put weight on.

In other words, there was a gulf between what I *thought* I ate, and what I *actually* ate on a daily basis.

I was very good at fooling myself; however, when I analysed my real food intake I was shocked at the amount of unnecessary food I would eat without noticing.

Does this sound familiar? I suspect that you are not much different from me!

For example, I used to eat low fat oven chips followed by a chocolate bar for my evening meal. I would then say to myself 'I will not eat anything else for the rest of the evening'. If I was being really 'good' and 'self-controlled' I would cut out the chocolate bar for a few days or sometimes even longer.

Yet when I stood on the scales I would be horrified by the fact that I had put weight on. Not only was I horrified, I was also shocked, because I had been so 'good' and cut out my evening chocolate bar.

I also would eat different types of food and not take a conscious note of the food – or perhaps I deluded myself by blocking these foods out from my conscious mind. It was only when I actually completed an honest analysis of my eating habits that I realised that I was in fact a 'secret eater'.

When I finally analysed my eating habits in an open, honest and accurate way, I was shocked by the amount of chocolate bars I would eat in one day without actually realising it.

I always brought a chocolate bar into work to eat at morning tea-break. I would sometimes have a biscuit – or three – at various times of the day – also without taking a mental note and adding this extra food to my perception of my daily food intake. On my way home from work I would often call into a newsagent's shop and buy a newspaper and another chocolate bar without thinking about it or adding it to the mental list of food I was eating that day (I was good at deluding myself – as are most secret eaters).

This was not the end of my secret eating as I would eat biscuits or another chocolate bar after my evening meal which I had eaten in a very fast manner (thus missing the signal from my stomach that I was full and should stop eating). Then, as I said already, I would say that that I would not eat anything else for the rest of the night and thought that I was being 'good'.

One of the problems was this was not the end of my eating for the night. I would settle to watch TV and would snack, once again, without mentally adding this food intake into my perceived calorie intake for the day.

I was not only fooling myself about the amount of food I was eating, I was also deluding myself about the *quality* of the food I was eating. In other words, I was eating more junk food than I was admitting to myself. I would say to myself 'I don't eat that badly'; however, when I stood on the scales I would wonder why I was so overweight despite the fact I did eat quite 'healthily'. I would take some healthy food and delude myself that I was eating well because I was blocking out the junk foods that I was eating. I was a secret eater in respect to the amount of junk that I was eating!

Being a 'secret eater' was a major problem and contributed to my obesity.

Fortunately I 'saw the light' and found the real, natural and long-lasting way to get fit and healthy. I did it and so can you!

How do you know if you are a secret eater?

The simplest and best way is to keep a food diary. This does not need to be complicated. You can just buy a small and cheap notebook and use this as a food diary to record your eating habits.

Maybe you are thinking that you can't be bothered to write everything down and can remember everything that you eat. If you can do this, then that is ok – as long as you keep a good *accurate* mental record of all of the food that you eat and don't delude yourself into thinking that you eat less than you actually do. Personally I found that I was able to fool myself by trying to rely on my mental record.

If you putting on weight every time you stand on the bathroom scales, and you just can't understand why, in spite of the fact that you are telling yourself that you *'don't eat that all much'* or you *'eat healthy food'* , please be honest with yourself and record everything that you eat.

Just like me, you may be surprised at the gulf between what you *think* that you eat and what you *actually* eat. Remember, we are good at deluding ourselves!

The good news is that if you follow the 'Three Point Plan' for weight loss and management outlined in this book, you will find that you can deal with the problem of being a 'secret eater'.

Emotional Eaters (comfort eaters)

Are you an '*emotional eater'*? I was. Another well-known term for emotional eater is 'comfort eater'.

Have you had a bad day at work? Do you make yourself feel better by having a bun or chocolate bar? Do you go straight for the biscuit barrel when you have a row with someone? Maybe you are facing very challenging circumstances in your life. Do you use eating as a means of making yourself feel better?

If the answer to any of the above statements is yes, then you are an emotional eater (comfort eater).

Life can be really tough, unfair and difficult to face and problems can seem as if they are never going to end at times.

Also, our emotional wounds can run very deep and we turn to food to help us feel better and face the world.

We are all individuals who each face our own unique challenges and problems. The issues that you face can be deep and complicated dating back to your childhood, leaving you with deep self-esteem or confidence issues.

Or you may be in a specific situation or crisis in your life that is making you eat for comfort (such as a job you hate or relationship difficulties).

Perhaps comfort eating has just become the means by which you have learned to make yourself feel better when everyday life is not going your way.

Irrespective of the reason for your emotional/comfort eating, the practical result is the same – you have developed a *bad habit*, and this bad habit can contribute in a major way to you having difficulties with weight gain and weight management.

The result is that you have learned to associate eating with making yourself feel better when you are not happy! But remember: it is a bad habit you have *learned*, and you can *unlearn* it!

Here is a summary of some key questions to ask yourself if you suspect that you are an emotional/comfort eater. Do any of the following apply to you? Are you: stressed? not hungry but eat for the sake of eating? sad? angry? anxious? bored? lonely? unemployed? unhappy in your job? unhappy with your partner?

If the answer is yes, do you eat to make yourself feel better?

Let's take a deeper look

We will now look more deeply into the area of emotional/comfort eating. Think carefully about the questions listed above and be honest about the answer – are you an emotional eater /comfort eater?

Again, I speak from my own personal experience because many of the calories I consumed which contributed to my weight gain were as a result of 'emotional' (or 'comfort') eating.

Think a little deeper about a time when you have had a very bad day.

Perhaps it was in work and you have come home in a very bad mood, stressed out or feeling down because of the negative events of the day.

Or perhaps you have been at home looking after young and demanding children. You love them dearly; however, the demands of looking after them have taken its toll and you are tired, frustrated and feeling down.

What do you do to cheer yourself up?

Probably the same thing that I used to do – head for the cupboard for some chocolate biscuits or crisps, or to the fridge for some cheesecake, or the freezer for some ice cream. You then sit on your comfy sofa and eat these great tasting snacks.

It is not just what you eat but also the amount that you eat!

Typically, you will also eat a large amount of these comfort foods, perhaps eating them at a fast speed. In other words you will *binge* on the comfort food of choice.

After you have eaten the lot you feel much better for a while – the food has given you comfort because of the problems you have faced in your life that day. But the feeling of comfort really only lasts for a while. You will then start to feel guilty because you know that you have eaten too much of the wrong type of food.

If you are overweight you will then feel bad about yourself because you don't like being overweight and this becomes a cycle that starts to spiral or spin out of control and leads to more comfort eating.

Why do we turn to food for comfort when we have been emotionally upset? Furthermore, why do we turn to particular foods – usually the most unhealthy or with the highest calorie content? This question is even more relevant to those people who are overweight and who don't like being overweight. You know that this binge eating is only going to make you gain even more weight.

There are a number of basic answers. The general over-reaching reason is we have been conditioned into this bad habit. We can be conditioned out of this habit, or perhaps I should say we can be re-educated to form better eating habits for pleasure that is consistent with the healthy way Nature intended.

Question: Is it always wrong to eat for comfort?

Answer: Of course not – there are times when emotional eating (comfort eating) is a good thing; however, there is a *wrong* way to comfort eat and a *right* way to comfort eat.

The wrong way and the right way

Remember the hunger pathways – Homeostatic (eating for need) and Hedonic (eating for pleasure). We have been genetically designed to enjoy food as evidenced by the fact that we have the Hedonic appetite (eating for pleasure) pathway alongside our vital for life Homeostatic (eating to fuel our bodies) appetite pathway.

So eating for pleasure is in itself not bad – in fact, it is a natural part of how we have been created.

However, the key phrase is *'balance'*. The Hedonic (eating for pleasure) is meant to supplement and support the Homeostatic (eating for need) appetite pathway. It is meant to be the servant, not the master.

When we comfort eat, we are overusing the Hedonic (pleasure) appetite pathway. Why do we do this? It is because we have allowed ourselves to get into the bad habit of doing so.

This goes hand in hand with overeating. We miss the natural signal telling us when we are hungry and when to stop. Remember Ghrelin and Leptin?

Ghrelin	Tells us that our body needs to eat to provide fuel for our body
Leptin	Tells us when we have had enough food (fuel)

How did we let ourselves be conditioned into the wrong way to comfort eat?

This is a complicated topic and there is no one simple answer; however, we will look at some important ideas which may help you to understand some of your reasons for emotional/comfort eating.

Let's go back to the very beginning. We will think back to when you were a baby. When you were hungry you followed your natural instincts and reflex to cry to alert the world to the fact that you needed to be fed.

The result of your cry was your mother fed you. This did two natural things – it satisfied your need to be fed and provided you with the comfort and security of having your needs met.

Fast forward to when you were a toddler. Remember those nice treats you got if you were fell and hurt your knees or when you recovered from an illness.

Fast forward again to when you were a couple of years older. Think back to the Saturday night family ice cream treat, or the special treat that your aunt or grandparents used to give you.

Remember those magical family Christmas holidays, when you got the presents that you were dreaming about, coupled with all of that lovely food that you scoffed.

Maybe you were given a much desired present for passing a certain set of exams or succeeding in a sporting event.

Associating food with good things, happy times and rewards which make us feel good has been deeply programmed into our subconscious mind.

Does this mean that using food as a celebration or comfort is wrong?

Absolutely not! Eating as part of a celebration or to cheer ourselves up is an essential part of human social interaction. The problem arises when we lose *perspective* of how to use food to celebrate or comfort ourselves.

Once we lose this perspective, bad habits contained within our *subconscious* mind dominate and control our eating habits.

The difference between our conscious and subconscious mind.

The conscious mind.

Neuro-scientists and psychologists tell us that we experience and deal with the everyday reality of our daily life in the world by means of our conscious mind.

The conscious mind is limited and can only deal with the world as it is in front of us in the immediate moment – that is what it is designed to do. We carry out our daily duties, make decisions, solve problems, and do our jobs, by concentrating with our conscious mind.

There is only so much that our conscious mind can deal with at one time. Once we move from one situation to another, the conscious mind needs to move on and deal with the new set of events in front of us. Psychologists call this movement an *'event boundary'*.

Event boundary.

Let me illustrate this: Have you ever left one room and gone into another to do something, only to find yourself standing there wondering what it is you have come into that room to do?

You will be standing there saying to yourself 'what did I come in here for?' You find yourself standing there at a loss as to what you had come into the room to do because your mind is a complete blank.

If you retrace your steps and go back to the room you have just left, you find that the thing you had entered the next room to do suddenly comes back to you, because you had gone back to the place you had first made the conscious decision to do what you needed to do in the next room.

You usually think to yourself that you are starting to lose your mind! No, you are not losing your mind or developing dementia if you do this on an occasional basis! We all do this. It is a symptom of dementia when it has become a major problem in the extent and frequency and is accompanied by other things which cause concern.

The reason why this happens is you have had an 'event boundary'. This means that your conscious mind has moved its focus from the room that you have just left and cleared itself in order to focus on the challenges of the new room you have just entered.

The reason why you forget what you wanted to do in the new room is the events from the old room have been 'filed away' into the subconscious mind so that you can use your conscious mind to focus on the immediate situation in front of you.

Remember, the conscious mind is limited and can only deal with so much at once.

The subconscious mind.

Unlike the conscious mind which is limited and only can deal with so much at a time, neuro-scientists and psychologists tell us that the subconscious mind is *unlimited* in what it can deal with and store. In fact, every sight, sound, smell and physical and emotional feeling you experienced throughout your entire life is stored in your subconscious mind.

Your subconscious mind is very powerful and it is largely responsible for the person you are and how you experience life.

Your confidence, self-esteem, academic achievement, relationship quality, views on life, behaviour and ***eating habits***, are all dictated and driven to a large degree by your subconscious mind.

It is important to remember that we store all of the things that we experience, including how events we experience make us *feel*! In other words, how we feel – good or bad, stay within our subconscious mind.

How do we bring the memories and feelings that are stored within our subconscious mind (sometimes very deeply) into our conscious mind? Also, how do the memories and feelings stored within our subconscious make us behave in the way we do, very often without us realising the impact of these deeply stored memories?

The answer to this question is complex; however, I am going to focus one of the key reasons – ***triggers!***

How often have you noticed a certain smell and all of a sudden you find yourself suddenly remembering a certain time from your past?

This can be so strong that you are almost transported back in time reliving the event associated with that smell. You say to yourself, 'Ah this takes me back' because everything comes flooding back to you.

It is not just smells that *trigger* this episode of reliving the past. It can be anything within all of the experiences of your whole life. It can be sounds, songs, colours, how a person looks, etc.

Significantly, we can relive some of the things stored deep within our subconscious mind without actually consciously realising it.

In other words, the subconscious mind influences how we behave and act, and we don't realise that this behaviour is happening as a result of *triggers* provoking the influence of our subconscious mind on how we act and behave.

Subconscious 'triggers' causing us to emotional/comfort eating.

Earlier we looked at how we associate food with happy events. These happy events and the nice food associated with them have been stored in the subconscious mind and led to the habit of associating the eating nice things with comfort or happy times.

This association is held within our subconscious and will surface in response to the appropriate trigger.

This in itself is not bad, in fact, this eating for comfort is actually *good and natural* if kept in *balance*.

However, with all of us who have engaged in emotional/comfort eating, somewhere along the line the positive aspects of the association of food with comfort and making ourselves feel good somehow became distorted and blown out of proportion. Perhaps we could say the servant became the master.

Now we must follow the *natural* way to re-educate our negative eating habits. The servant must be removed from the elevated position of being the master and back to its natural role of servant. It is important to comfort eat, but in the correct way.

How can we bring our emotional (comfort) eating under control?

Please note that I did not ask the question: *how can we stop emotional eating?*

Remember, we are created and designed to *enjoy* and get *pleasure* from eating as well as eating to stay alive - remember *Homeostatic* (eating to stay alive) and *Hedonic* (eating for pleasure). It is good to celebrate special occasions by eating a special meal to contribute to the feel good factor of the special occasion. Imagine how bland and joyless life would be if we did not enjoy those special treats!

It is also good *sometimes* to eat a specific food to cheer yourself up if you are feeling down and life is getting on top of you. Remember, you have been naturally programmed to get pleasure from eating, and at times it is right to use different things to help make us feel better when we are low.

The key thing is *balance*. It is natural to engage in emotional eating; however, is unnatural and unhealthy to let this type of eating grow to the point where you are controlled by comfort eating. When this happens you have moved from using food in a positive way, to letting it control you and lead to you becoming an 'emotional eater'

Using food in the correct way to help with times of emotion (both positive and negative times) is a good and natural thing to do, but using it as a tool to deal with the difficult times feelings and situations will contribute to our weight gain.

Here are some practical suggestions to help you deal with your bad habit of emotional eating. These strategies may help you deal with emotional eating habits.

Know and understand the difference between emotional/comfort eating hunger and true hunger in your stomach (tummy hunger).

In order to re-educate yourself to change the habit of emotional/comfort eating, you must understand and remember difference between emotional hunger (a type of 'head hunger') and true hunger in your stomach ('tummy hunger').

Emotional/comfort eating is a form of 'head hunger' which leads us to eat when we don't need to fuel our body with food. In fact, it is a very powerful form of 'head hunger', and one that can be hard to move away from as it involves deep-seated and sometimes powerful feelings and emotions.

Question: *'How can we tell the difference between true physical hunger ('tummy hunger') and false emotional hunger (a type of 'head hunger')?*

This is an important question and when you understand the difference, you will have made a major step forward in your battle to achieve and maintain your ideal healthy weight.

Emotional hunger (the desire to comfort eat) always hits you ***suddenly***.

In contrast, true physical hunger (tummy hunger) is a feeling that builds *gradually*.

Emotional hunger will usually result in the strong desire to eat certain very ***specific foods items you associate with comfort.***

You will strongly crave very sugary or fatty foods that will give you the instant rush you desire to make yourself feel better. You will strongly feel that you really *need* one of the following examples of common comfort foods: cheesecake, pizza, chocolate cake, large bag of crisps, large portion of chips (French fries), a whole packet of chocolate biscuits (cookies), etc.

Emotional eating often results in ***thoughtless*** eating without any conscious thoughts or regards about the amount that you are actually eating. Once you open the packet of biscuits or cookies (or whatever your comfort food happens to be), you find that you have eaten the whole packet before you know it.

Emotional hunger does ***not make you feel full or satisfied.*** This leads on from the previous point. Once you have finished your thoughtless eating and find that the packet of your comfort food of choice is finished, you will not be satisfied and still want to eat more – you really are 'on a roll' when it comes to comfort eating and just want to eat more and more.

Emotional hunger is ***not true 'tummy hunger'*** – it does not begin gradually in the *stomach* area, in the way true hunger does.

If you eat in response to emotional hunger as opposed to true stomach hunger, you will usually regret the fact that you have just eaten an entire packet of cookies (or whatever your comfort food actually is) and so end up with feelings of *guilt* and *shame***.** This is because you know that you didn't actually need that food. This feeling is worse if you are overweight because you know that you have just contributed to that fact that you will continue to be trapped in the 'prison' of being overweight, and this will make you feel bad about yourself.

Remember, emotional eating is usually in response to ***triggers***!

As we have already looked at in this chapter, the things stored in our subconscious affect our behaviour in response to triggers. Certain events will trigger our desire to eat to make ourselves feel better. Emotional eating can be triggered by the emotions associated with both negative and unpleasant experiences (stress, etc) and positive and pleasant experience (the desire to reward yourself for achieving a key goal in life or enjoying a holiday or Christmas memories, etc).

Here is a summary of the main differences between emotional/comfort eating and true tummy hunger:

Emotional Hunger	**True physical (tummy) hunger**
The desire to comfort eat will hit you *suddenly*.	The true desire to eat in order to provide your body with fuel to stay alive will build *slowly*.
This desire to comfort eat will be as a result of a negative 'trigger' in your life (stress, work problems, relationship difficulties, etc).	True tummy hunger will grow gradually as a result of your body releasing signals when you need to put food into your body to stay alive.
The desire to comfort eat will demand instant satisfaction.	True physical hunger will be able to wait until the gradual feeling of true hunger becomes overwhelming.
When you comfort eat you will usually crave your favourite specific comfort foods.	When you are truly tummy hungry, you will be happy to eat a variety of foods. In fact, you will want to have a 'nice dinner' with a balance of food types.
When you comfort eat, you do not know when to stop eating. You will keep eating until your stomach is full; however, your hunger will not feel satisfied because it is emotional hunger.	When you are truly tummy hungry, you will stop eating when you are full (if you are following the 'Three Point Plan' and eating the way you have been designed to do).
When you comfort eat, you will feel bad about yourself, especially if you are overweight. You will feel guilty and ashamed.	When you eat to satisfy true tummy hunger, you will not have any negative feeling about yourself as you know that you are eating in response to a natural process required to keep to you alive.

Be honest with yourself

Be honest with yourself and recognise that you are using foods in the wrong way to make yourself feel better.

Remember that it is a bad habit.

You were not born as an emotional eater; rather, you have been conditioned at various times of your life into the bad habit of turning to food for comfort. If you have been conditioned into this bad habit, then you can be conditioned out of this bad habit.

Follow the *'Three Point Plan'* for weight loss outlined in this book to re-educate your eating habits. If you stick to the principle of *only eating when you are really hungry in your stomach ('tummy hungry')*, then you will not comfort eat.

When you do start to comfort eat, if you stick to the second point of the 'Three point Plan' (*eat slowly),* you will reduce the amount of food that you eat. This will help you control your weight and reduce the feelings of guilt, as you will have the feeling of being more in control.

Substitute a healthy alternative

If you really must eat, then use an alternative natural snack food that will not pile on the pounds. If you follow the 'Three Point Plan', you will not eat too much.

Drink a glass of water

We can mistake hunger for thirst. If we have a strong desire to eat, sometimes we can bring this desire to an end by taking a glass of water. It is worth a try.

Learn to control your cravings

Please read the chapter 'Cravings – the enemy of weight loss'. This chapter will give you some practical tips on how control your cravings. Emotional/comfort eating is more than just a craving for a particular food; however, the practical tips are relevant and can be applied with good effect when you are craving a particular food to make yourself feel better.

Allow yourself to comfort eat occasionally.

Let's use the illustration of a healthy bank balance.

If you have a healthy bank balance and you are 'in the black', then you can afford to occasionally spend money on superficial things that you don't really need without worry or guilt. On the other hand, if you spend money on such things and you don't have a healthy bank balance (you are 'in the red'), then you cannot justify spending and wasting money on these unnecessary things.

Furthermore, you could find yourself in real trouble. You will find yourself moving from being in the 'black' to being in the 'red' if you don't control your superficial spending – it is only fine if you do it occasionally.

The same is true of eating. If you are eating in the way you have been designed to do and managing your weight naturally (by following the 'Three Point Plan'), then you can afford to occasionally indulge in comfort eating without any real damage being done to your weight management – you can 'afford' it without feeling guilty.

On the other hand, if you are struggling with your weight, you cannot 'afford' to indulge in unnecessary eating habits. It will make your weight problem worse and provoke negative feelings of guilt, etc.

If you have achieved and are maintaining your ideal healthy weight by following the 'Three Point Plan', then your body's fantastic waste removal system will deal with the food contents of the occasional unnecessary and unhealthy eating episode – such as the occasional indulgence in comfort eating.

On the other hand, if you overload the waste disposal system of your body with too much unnecessary food it will stop dealing with it efficiently by passing it out of your body, and will be forced to store the excess as fat. This is the very thing that you want to avoid.

Keep a diary or journal of your emotional/comfort eating.

An excellent way to help you identify any patterns to your emotional eating habits is to keep an emotional/comfort eating diary or journal.

Perhaps you don't like the thought of keeping a written record of your emotional/comfort eating habits. You may automatically think that you don't have the time to sit and write a diary, or that you really can't be bothered with the hassle.

You don't need to create a complicated or elaborate emotional eating diary requiring a lot of writing. All you need is a simple template with minimal writing, providing you with an effective record of the patterns of your emotional eating habits.

The insights you notice about the patterns of your negative emotional eating habits may be useful and help you deal more effectively with this particular problem.

Develop healthy lifestyle habits.

You can make a big difference to your ability to deal with difficult times without turning to food for comfort.

It can be useful for you do make time for a specific *relaxation* session of at least 30 minutes. If your automatic reaction to this is you are 'far too busy' and have 'too much to do' and can't afford to take 30 minutes off to relax – this is proof that you really *do* need to take the time out of your stress filled day in order to unwind and 'recharge your batteries'

Do some physical activity or exercise.

Exercise and physical activity can really help you reduce the effects of stress and boost your mood when you are under emotional attack. Please don't let the thought of physical activity or exercise create a negative reaction in your mind. I am not necessarily talking about 'hitting the gym' or 'pumping iron'.

Exercise is not just going to the gym or going for a run. You may be at the stage that you can go for a run and this will make you feel better. But don't worry if you are not at this fitness level at the moment.

Remember, exercise is anything that makes your heart beat faster and your lungs breathe more deeply. Therefore, exercise can be going for a brisk walk or doing everyday activities done with greater vigour, such as vacuuming the carpet or cutting the grass, etc.

It may be that your desire to use food to help yourself deal with the negative feelings of a stressful day can be replaced by a short bout of a physical activity which is appropriate to your personal fitness levels. Please read the chapter on 'Exercise'.

Know your triggers

What is the trigger that makes you want to comfort eat? This is a question that does not have a simple answer. There are many things that can trigger our desire to engage in emotional eating. However, if you can train yourself to recognise many of the events, situations or feeling which trigger your desire to comfort eat, you will be in a better position deal with your desire to comfort eat.

Let's look at the most common trigger:

Stress

I would suggest that stress is the most common reason for our ongoing emotional/comfort eating. We all suffer from stress as it is part of our everyday life in this fast moving world that we live in. We find ourselves daily in situations that cause us to become stressed.

We have to get up in the morning and get ourselves and possibly the kids up and dressed to face work and school. We then have to face the stress of the commute to work with all of the hassles that brings (traffic jams, crowded trains with rude people, icy roads, etc).

Maybe you are stressed because you *don't* work either through unemployment, retirement, child care, illness, etc.

Perhaps you hate your job because the workload is too much or you are bullied by a horrible boss. Maybe you have had an argument with your partner or parent. The list of things which can cause stress on a daily basis is almost never-ending.

Many of us have the bad habit of turning to food as a means of making ourselves feel better. In other words, we comfort eat to bring emotional relief.

What is stress?

We all face stress, but do we really fully understand what stress is and how it actually affects us?

You need stress to stay alive!

Yes, you have not misread this heading – you do need stress to stay alive. Stress is hot-wired into your DNA, or more accurately, the *stress response* has been hotwired into your DNA, which means that you have been genetically programmed to have the *stress response.* It is the stress response that keeps you alive and to function in the challenging and sometimes dangerous world in which we live.

Why do we need stress?

Time for an illustration: The stress response in our body is like a smoke detector fire alarm in a building or a car alarm in your vehicle. The purpose of these alarms is to detect and warn when there is something wrong. They are designed to protect you and prepare you to deal with danger.

Neuro-scientists and psychologists tell us that the stress response has a similar purpose in our body. It is part of our *'fight or flight'* response to danger.

The human body is truly remarkable and has been wonderfully designed. Think about all of the things that happens in our body without us even thinking about it. Your heart beats, your blood flows, your food passes through your body and the nutrients you need to stay alive are taken out, etc.

One of these automatic processes your body has been designed to perform is the 'fight or flight' response. This is not a just mental state or state of mind. Rather, it is a *physical* response in your *brain* which leads to both *mental* and *physical* reactions.

The part of the brain responsible for controlling this is the *limbic system.* In addition to 'fight or flight', this system is involved in other key functions such as the regulation and processing of emotions and long-term memories.

It includes the following structures: *amygdala* (emotion centre); *hippocampus* (long term-memory formation); *thalamus* (relaying sensory and motor signals from the 'unconscious' to the 'conscious' and 'thought processing' area of the brain); *hypothalamus* (controls hormone release); *cingulate gyrus* (regulates and coordinates smells and sights with pleasant memories, emotional reaction to pain, flexibility and adaptability).

All of the information gathered from your senses and sent to your brain is received and processed at a *subconscious* level by the limbic system, before it is passed on to the relevant parts of the brain for you to take action and respond at a *conscious* level.

One key role of the limbic system is to keep you alive, safe and happy. In order to do this, it will process and interpret all incoming information from our senses and help us decide of the situation we are faced with is good for our health, safety and well-being.

If the limbic system decides that a situation is not good for our physical or mental well-being, it will direct our mind and body to react in a way that will make us safe or feel better.

Remember, this all happens at a *subconscious* level; however, it will produce real mental and physical responses in our body.

Appropriate stress is good and will produce positive reactions in our body - enabling us to continue in and deal with a difficult situation, or leave.

However, too much stress can result in negative responses in our body, such as headaches, frequent colds, stomach problems, skin conditions, etc.

Long term, too much of the stress chemical *cortisol* will weaken muscle and bones, and can shorten life expectancy for up to five years or more.

The stress response is not weakness – it is part of your genetic programming. You can't just 'snap out of it' or 'pull yourself together'.

On the contrary, we must understand and work with the stress response. Failure to do so can result in major problems for you physical and mental health.

The 'fight or flight' response will lead you to subconsciously draw upon a number of strategies. You have learned and stored away these strategies to be called upon to help you deal with the situation causing your stress levels to rise. One of these subconscious strategies can be *comfort eating.*

You have been gradually conditioned to form the habit comfort eating. To deal effectively with this problem, you need to gradually re-educate yourself away from this bad habit. This cannot be achieved by dieting and will-power. It can be achieved by following the 'Three Point Plan'.

Let's think about the 'fight or flight' response:

Remember, this is actually a physical response in your brain which leads to both physical and emotional reactions in your mind and body!

It works something like this: Suppose you were walking along a street and someone jumped out of an alleyway and threatened you with a gun or knife or an aggressive dog ran at you barking and showing its teeth. Your body would automatically go into the '*stress response'* (you would rightly become stressed) which would result in our brain automatically directing number of chemical and physical reactions in our body.

Your body would start to pump ***cortisol*** (the stress hormone) and *adrenaline* into your system to help you survive this situation. Your heart rate would dramatically increase to pump extra blood and oxygen into the muscles of your arms and legs to provide you with extra energy to either run (flight) or defend yourself (fight) from the danger in front of you. We need this stress response otherwise we would not live very long as we would not be able to deal with the threats and dangers we all face.

This system is fantastic when it functions in the correct circumstances (such as when you face a real danger) and its application is appropriate and proportional to the situation and threat you find yourself facing. However, a problem arises when this system operates at a level which is not appropriate to help keep you alive.

Let me explain this further. I have talked about how the body creates a stress response to a physical threat that you may find yourself facing. However, neuro-scientists and psychologists tell us that the body cannot tell the difference between a '*real physical*' threat and a '*psychological or imagined'* threat.

Real physical threat and psychological or imagined threat.

When someone pulls out a gun or knife and points it at you, or an aggressive dog comes running at you, these are *real* threats – you could get seriously injured or lose your life. When someone is critical of you or you cannot meet a deadline and cope with the workload at work, or when you have a major row and disagreement with your spouse, partner or parent, these are *psychological or imagined* threats.

Psychological or imagined threats will create the same stress responses as real threats - your body cannot tell the difference. This means that stressful situations in home, relationships, work, school, etc, have a real physical effect on your body and your mind.

We naturally do not like these effects of stress, and many of us have learned the bad habit of turning to food to help get rid of these unpleasant effects and make ourselves feel better.

It is vital from a weight management point of view to understand this and take the steps outlined earlier to deal with emotional eating.

We can also learn to develop better strategies for dealing with and controlling the effects of stress without food when we understand what is going on.

There are plenty of self-help books and websites out there which can help you develop better ways to deal with your stress. Please don't hesitate to see your family doctor for help if stress is becoming too much for you.

Other triggers include:

Boredom

If you are bored, eating can provide you with something to do. Please be aware of this and ask yourself if you are about to eat because you are truly hungry in your stomach (tummy hungry) or eating because you are bored. If it is because you are bored, please be creative and find something else to fill your time and deal with your boredom. There is always something constructive to do if you give it enough thought.

Loneliness

We humans are social beings and we need other human beings. Admittedly, some of us will need more social interaction with other people than others depending on our personality; however, we all do need other people.

When we don't get our natural need for meaningful companionship satisfied, we can suffer from the powerful negative emotion of loneliness.

Loneliness is not the same as being alone. You can be alone for long periods of time and not be lonely. Alternatively, you can be in a crowded room and feel very lonely because you don't feel that you 'fit in' with the people present in a real and meaningful way.

Loneliness is a very powerful negative emotion, which causes the lonely person to experience very unpleasant feelings.

It is very tempting to lapse into the bad habit of emotional/comfort eating to try to make yourself feel better.

If you are feeling lonely and feel the urge to eat, please take the time to work out if it is true physical hunger or emotional hunger.

Many other things.

I cannot hope to list all of the things in life that can trigger the negative bad habit of turning to food as a way of making ourselves feel better. Life is challenging and unfair at times. It is not always possible even to imagine or foresee some of the things that may happen in our life until they actually happen.

One thing we can be sure of is that we will face times of emotional difficulty.

We can't stop the negative things that life will throw at us; however, we can move away from being dominated by the bad habit of turning to food to make us feel better by comfort eating.

The key point to remember about emotional/comfort eating:

If you are an emotional eater, you will find yourself being tempted by emotional hunger to make yourself feel better in negative situations. However, when you do find yourself heading to the cupboard or fridge to find your comfort food of choice, please make sure that you use the tips outlined in this chapter to help you avoid emotional/comfort eating.

Habit Eaters

Are you a '*habit eater*'?

Eating out of habit was probably one of the faulty eating habits that led to the biggest contribution to my weight gain and ongoing struggle with losing weight

What do I mean by eating out of habit? Think about this example:

It is mid-morning tea-time in work or in the house. You make yourself a cup of tea or coffee. The tea is nice; however, you must also have a biscuit or something sweet with your drink otherwise you say 'It just doesn't taste the same'.

Or perhaps after your evening meal you must have a particular chocolate bar or dessert. Do you look for a packet of crisps or sweet thing as you are watching TV in the evening or feel that you can't really enjoy a movie at the cinema without a king-size carton of popcorn?

Why? The answer is very simple – you have formed the habit of eating biscuits with certain hot drinks or after certain meals.

You have been conditioned into looking for the biscuits, crisps, popcorn etc, at certain points or moments of time. It is a habit that you have formed. The good news is that this bad habit can be replaced by better eating habits.

This cannot be done by dieting.

It can be achieved long term and permanently by changing how you think about food and eating by using the techniques I have been describing in this book.

I was a habit eater and this habit eating contributed in a major way to my obesity. I loved to munch as I watched TV or movies, etc. I also used to eat biscuits and chocolate bars at times when I did not need them. I dread to thing how many calories I consumed just by habit-eating alone.

Thankfully, I became aware of the problem of *habit-eating*. This awareness is an important factor in my permanent weight loss.

Once I was aware of this problem, I was able to work out a way of controlling my negative practice of habit-eating in a natural and permanent way.

How do you do it?

Basically, you will use the same techniques outlined in the previous chapter on emotional and comfort eating.

Forget the dieting and willpower and use the following techniques and principles.

Follow the 'Three Pint Plan' to help you form good eating habits, which are based on the principles found in Nature, to ensure that we eat the way our bodies have been genetically designed to do.

Read and follow processes outlined in the chapter 'Cravings, the enemy of weight loss'. If you must eat during a movie, consider substituting healthier snack options. Keep popcorn for the occasional trip to the cinema.

If you follow the above techniques you will stop or reduce your habit eating enough to make a difference to your weight management and you will achieve the ideal weight for you.

Habits

Throughout this book I have repeatedly used the word habit. In fact, the concept of habit is central to our understanding of both how we put on weight, and crucially, how we can lose and manage our weight on a permanent basis. Put in its most basic terms: We gain weight by means of developing bad eating habits. On the other hand, we lose weight by re-educating ourselves to replace these bad eating habits with good eating habits.

What is a habit?

According to neuro-science and psychology, a habit is a learned behaviour that a person repeats on a regular basis until he or she continues to do it without thinking consciously about it. This repeated behaviour often happens without the person noticing that they are developing the habit. Research suggests that it takes about sixty-six days for behaviour to become a habit for most people. Remember, once a particular behaviour becomes a habit, we engage in that behaviour without thinking about it or realising that we are doing it.

Our eating patterns are habits, and the size of our waistline and quality of our health will be dictated by whether we have good natural eating habits, or bad unnatural ones.

Once a habit has become established, it is hard to break, and the deeper and more ingrained in us the habit, the more difficult it is to break. This is because the habit becomes imprinted into the *neural pathways* in our brain and deeply into our subconscious.

It is impossible for most people to break a strongly or deeply established habit using willpower because you *cannot change the neural pathways in your brain with willpower alone*!

The only way to break a deeply established habit is to gradually replace it with a more appropriate habit. This will require focus and effort, but it is easier than trying to use willpower to stick to a diet.

In other words, you need to change the behaviour programmed into the neural pathways in your brain, by gradually developing new neural pathways. This change to the neural pathways cannot be done by diets or willpower!

This is one of the reasons why most diets do not result in permanent weight loss. Once you come off the diet, you slip back into your old eating habits and regain the weight. It can, however, be achieved by following the principles outlined in this book.

Chapter 14

Cravings – the enemy of weight loss

Do you know what it is like to crave a certain food item? I certainly do, and I can say with confidence that anyone who is struggling with their weight will know the full force of the power of cravings.

Cravings are one of the biggest enemies of weight loss and weight management. You will know how many times you have been annoyed at yourself because you have been trying to lose weight, but just could not resist the overwhelming craving for that chocolate bar, chocolate cake, cheesecake, packet of cookies, or whatever your particular desired food item happens to be.

The good news is cravings can be controlled, and you can do this without giving up those items of food that you crave so much. Yes, that is correct, you can eat those nice goodies that you love so much; however, the key is being able to control *when* you eat these treats, and the *amount.*

A craving is another *bad habit* that controls us and we become the servant of the craving. We can learn to break the power of the craving, and control ourselves when faced with it.

Craving is a type of *imagined* hunger (*'head hunger'),* not *true physical hunger in the stomach ('tummy hunger').* We have looked at the difference between head hunger and tummy hunger and how crucial it is for weight loss to understand the difference.

When we are hit with a craving, we usually desire a particular food (usually one full of sugar or unhealthy fats). It will come on us very *suddenly* and very *powerfully*, and we will want to satisfy it *immediately*.

Remember, in contrast, true hunger in the stomach ('tummy hunger') is a *gradual* sensation which is satisfied when we take in the fuel we need – as long as we are following natural eating principles, such as those outlined in this book!

The processes associated with cravings are very similar to those involved in 'emotional eating' habits and we use some of the same strategies to overcome both. However, cravings may require some additional strategies and we will look at some of these shortly.

I will now outline some of the strategies I used to help beat my cravings.

Remember that it is a bad habit.

In the same way that you were not born as an emotional or habit eater, you were not born to have cravings. Rather, you have been conditioned at various times of your life into the bad habit of turning to food in an inappropriate way. If you have been conditioned into this bad habit, then you can be conditioned out of this bad habit.

Follow the 'Three Point Plan' for weight loss to control your hunger

1. Eat only when you are genuinely hungry - in your stomach, not your imagination (or 'tummy hungry' to use the old well known phrase).

Learn to 'listen' to your body when it releases the hunger hormone (Ghrelin), to let you know it is time to eat and 're-fuel' your body with food.

2. Eat slowly and enjoy each mouthful.

Slow down, chew your food slowly and do not scoff the food down – as you may have told when you were a child.

3. Stop eating when you feel that your stomach feels full.

Learn to 'listen' to your body when it naturally sends the chemical (Leptin) to let you know your stomach it is full.

If you establish the correct eating patterns as outlined in this book, you will find that you will not be hungry all the time, in the way that you probably are now if you are overweight. I well remember this feeling of constant hunger.

If you are not hungry, then you will be less likely to crave certain foods. This is because you have re-educated yourself to stick to the 'Three Point Plan', especially the principle of *only eating when you are hungry in your stomach (tummy hungry).*

Just wait, stand firm and see if the craving passes.

Willpower is useless when it comes to resisting food; however, that is not to say that at times it does not have its place.

Sometimes, especially if the craving is not too strong, you will be able to resist and the notion will wear off. If not, then use some of the following strategies.

Distract yourself.

A wise man once told me about an old saying which I think can be applied to dealing with a craving. The man was talking in a different context from food; however, the principle is relevant and can be applied to food craving. He was in fact talking about people battling alcohol addiction.

The saying is:

'If you want a drink, go polish your shoes'.

This gentleman had a problem with drink in the past, to the point where he had to face the fact that he had become an alcoholic. Thankfully he won his battle with alcohol and put his life back on track with a good job, nice home, etc.

He has not had a drink for well over thirty years; however, he is very aware that there is always a danger that alcohol could take hold of him again, if he let it.

The gentleman uses this old saying very effectively if he feels himself being tempted to have a drink. In the early days especially, he would distract himself by doing something else, such as polishing his shoes! He now passes this advice on to other people who may be struggling to resist a drink.

The craving for food is not quite the same thing, and not as difficult to deal with as an addiction to alcohol; however, the principle is the same. Remember, change the words of this old wise saying to:

'If you crave a food item, go polish your shoes'.

Try the 'Swap Technique' (substitute 'disgusting' for 'pleasure' principle)

We crave certain foods because we associate pleasure with them – we really like them. On the other hand, we also avoid certain foods because we find them disgusting and really dislike them. We don't crave foods that we do not like!

How come we love certain foods and hate others?

Let's think about this in more detail.

Foods we like.

We eat certain foods because we like the taste and the effect it has on us. Chocolate is a prime example.

Do you consider yourself to be addicted to chocolate (a chocoholic)? I know I certainly would have considered myself addicted to chocolate. I just couldn't get enough of the stuff. The craving for chocolate would hit me many times during the day.

Why was this? Simple answer – I loved the taste of chocolate and the taste made me feel good. All of the ingredients contained in chocolate had a positive effect on my brain.

The result was I created a positive association of pleasure with chocolate. So when I saw a chocolate bar, it provoked these positive associations and I just wanted to eat chocolate.

Food we hate.

Think of the foods you hate. Why do you hate these foods?

More specifically, is there a particular food that makes you feel sick, even of you just think about it?

Why is this?

It is probably because you have had a negative experience with the food item in question. Perhaps it gave you a tummy ache, made you physically throw up or gave you diarrhoea. Even worse, you may even have become very ill through food poisoning.

How do you feel when you are faced with that food item which made you sick? You will avoid that food because your subconscious has been conditioned to avoid it. One thing is certain – you will not crave that particular food item.

What if you could learn to swap these associations?

In other words, if you could learn to swap the feelings of desire you have for the item you crave for the feelings of disgust for the food you avoid, you will stop your cravings.

I am now going to outline the technique for you. I have found it helpful and hopefully you will too. It will not work for everybody, but it is worth a try.

The technique works something like this:

Think of the food you crave.

Think of a food that disgusts you.

Swap these in your head and imaging that the food you love tastes like the food you hate.

If you concentrate hard and apply this technique when you are looking at a food item and craving it, you may find that this will help you lose the craving for that food item.

Take a drink of water.

We can mistake hunger for thirst. If we have a strong desire to eat, sometimes we can bring this desire to an end by taking a glass of water. It is worth a try.

Set aside a specific time to indulge your craving

A little of what you fancy is ok. This applies to chocolate, cheesecake, cookies or whatever food types you crave.

Remember, we are designed and programmed to enjoy eating (the Hedonic or 'eating for pleasure' appetite pathway) as long as pleasure eating is the servant and not the master!

I set aside specific days during the week (usually Saturday or Sunday) when I will enjoy a lovely big bar of chocolate or a cheesecake, etc.

If I find myself wanting to eat chocolate during week days, I will remind myself to look forward to the Saturday treat. More often than not this is now enough to move away from looking at that chocolate bar.

Occasionally, the desire is very strong, so I use the 'Swap Technique' outlined earlier in the chapter. I am delighted to say that for me, the cravings are nowhere near as powerful as they used to be.

A little of what you fancy

I used to call myself a chocoholic because I craved chocolate almost constantly. But I wasn't a chocoholic! I know now that my craving for chocolate was a bad *habit* established through faulty conditioning.

I am glad to say that I have changed this habit and don't crave chocolate now to the same level. However;

there are occasions when I do have a strong desire for some chocolate.

In addition to some of the techniques outlined above, I sometimes use a very simple technique where I will buy a small bar of children's chocolate and eat it slowly and let the chocolate melt in my mouth. This satisfies my desire for the taste of chocolate without actually doing any damage to my waistline. Sometimes I follow this by chewing some gum to trick my brain, because my jaws are moving as if I were eating.

Make yourself a healthy homemade milkshake.

If you really fancy the taste of something with a chocolate or similar sweet taste you could make yourself a simple and healthy milkshake.

All you need is half a pint of milk (skimmed or semi-skimmed), 1 teaspoonful of drinking chocolate and either a blender or a sports 'shaker bottle' (available very cheaply from sports stores). Simply add your teaspoon of drinking chocolate to the cold milk, blend (or shake in your sports shaker bottle if you don't have a blender) and enjoy.

Please note that this is this option should only be followed occasionally. You should follow the other options outlined in this chapter first, as it is better to beat the craving.

Chapter 15

Do you drink enough water?

One of the key principles emphasised during my studies to become a qualified Fitness Instructor was the importance of *hydration* – drinking enough water!

This principle of drinking enough water applies both to exercise programmes and to our daily life, and leads to the important question:

Do *you* drink enough water every day?

Did you know that drinking a glass of water can actually help you lose weight?

Yes, that is correct – I am talking about an ordinary glass of drinking water from your kitchen tap or faucet, water cooler in work or bottle of water.

Question: How can a glass of water help us lose weight - does it burn calories and fat?

Answer: The answer of course is no!

Let me explain how the glass of water helps us in our weight management programme.

You can mistake thirst for hunger!

If you understand this principle, then you will have an important tool in your weight management 'tool box'.

We all know that water is vital to life. It is possible to live longer without food that it is to live without water.

Our body is made up of 75% water, and our brain is genetically programmed to make sure that the water we put into our body is distributed in correct proportion to the internal organs. Therefore, it is essential to make sure we drink enough water ever day if this is going to be done with the efficiency required for maximum health.

Many of us are dehydrated and don't even know it.

How does our brain make sure that we have enough water? The simple and obvious answer is that it makes us *thirsty!*

Thirst and hunger do similar jobs. When we need food to fuel our body, our brain sends a signal that we are hungry and need to eat food. Similarly, when we need water to be distributed to our body, our brain sends a signal that we are thirsty and need to drink water.

Question: What has this got do with weight loss?

Answer: We can mistake the thirst signal to drink for the hunger signal to eat.

Keep this in mind when you feel a strong desire to eat and ask yourself, *'Am I hungry or thirsty'*?

You should then go and drink a glass of water and wait to see if the desire to eat goes away. If it does, then you have mistaken thirst for hunger.

Water obviously keeps us alive, and it is essential to maintain the body fluids balance. However, there are many health and fitness reasons why we should make sure we drink enough water every day.

Chapter 16

Exercise

I am finding the writing of this chapter very exciting from a personal point of view. An important part of my weight loss journey was my effort to get fit again. Not only did I achieve a fitness level far beyond anything I dared to imagine back in my days of obesity, I am amazed and delighted with the fact that I have trained and qualified as a professional Fitness Instructor.

This means that I am writing this chapter about exercise both from my experience of getting fit as part of my weight loss and from the professional point of view as a qualified Fitness Instructor.

Let's think about the word *exercise*.

Think for a moment about a TV show or a movie where you see a psychologist playing a game of word association with a patient. The psychologist says a word and the patient says what they associate with that word. For example, the word may be 'sky' and the patient may say '*cloud*' or '*bird*'.

We are now going to play a game of word association.

I am going to say a word and I want you to think about it and say out loud the first thing that you associate with this word.

The word is: '*Exercise*'.

Be honest, what did you think about and associate with this word? Was it a negative association? Was it one or more of the following?

The gym.
Pumping iron.
Treadmills.
Rowing Machines.
Exercise bikes.
Sweat.
Exhaustion.
Being shouted at in an exercise class.
Lycra gym outfits you feel too self-conscious to wear.
Embarrassment.
Posers with muscles.

The list of possible negative associations that you may have with the word exercise goes on and on.

Maybe you have very bad memories of being embarrassed in school in PE classes. Or maybe you used to enjoy PE and physical activities, but over the years you have 'let yourself go' and have gradually become an overweight couch potato. I must be honest and say that I fall into the latter category. I enjoyed PE and games at school, and was active until I hit my mid-twenties, then the gradual decline towards becoming an overweight and inactive couch potato began. It didn't happen overnight – it was a slow process.

Please do not let yourself be put off by the word 'exercise'. It has a negative effect on a lot of people and can also be very scary to someone who currently wants to lose weight. I know because I was one of those people. I really wanted to be fit again; however, the four and a half stone of excess weight I was carrying around, and the breathlessness I experienced after walking up a hill or stairs, was a constant reminder of just how unfit I was. I was on medication for high cholesterol and high blood pressure.

It was clear to me that I was going to need to do some form of exercise. I decided to follow a programme that guided me through a gradual step-by-step programme.

I was an unfit couch potato, even though I did try to kid myself that I did walk when I could. I did not walk as much as I should to make any difference to my fitness level.

I am glad to say that I have achieved a very high fitness level – much higher than I could have imagined back when I was four and a half stone overweight. I even completed a half-marathon Also, as already mentioned, I am now a qualified Fitness Instructor.

Why do a lot of people (I gradually became one of them) react so negatively to the word 'exercise'?

The main reason is we have become conditioned to react this way.

Here are two of the main reasons:

- We do not associate the word exercise with pleasure.
- We confuse the concept of *exercise* with *exercise programmes*.

Let's look a little bit deeper at these concepts.

We don't associate exercise with pleasure.

Maybe you do not associate the word exercise with pleasure - quite the reverse in fact. Rather, you think about hard workouts with tough talking Fitness Instructors who will push you until you are soaked in sweat and sore all over, and made to feel like an inadequate failure.

Or, maybe you feel too unfit and too embarrassed to face the fit gym users (I know that I did).

Maybe you have persuaded yourself that you are too old. Perhaps you have health problems and think exercise is just a non-starter, etc.

It is vital that you stop thinking about exercise being a negative thing.

When you start seeing exercise for what it really is, this will help you discover the joy of exercise and will become a natural part of your life.

The difference between 'exercise' and 'exercise programmes'.

We must understand the difference between *exercise* and *exercise programmes*. Once you do understand the difference, it will transform your attitude to exercise, and will prove to be a real game changer in terms of your new healthy lifestyle. It goes with the weight loss and weight management programme just as a horse and carriage go together.

Summary the ***difference*** between ***exercise & exercise programmes*** (I will expand on this later in the chapter):

Exercise	Your everyday activities. Anything that means you move your body and make your heart beat more quickly and lungs breathe more deeply. These things are exercise - you just need to recognise this. The basis of your new exercise attitude and programme is doing these things which you do every day, and just do them with more effort. This is your: *'Level A' or ongoing /foundation everyday fitness'.*	Walking up stairs. Carrying your shopping. Vacuuming your carpet. Mowing the lawn. Hanging out the washing. Walking the dog.
Exercise programmes	Specific activities tailored and designed to give you a specific workout over and above your normal daily routines and activities. This is your: *'Level B' or extra/add on activities'* that you add on to your fitness programme.	Going to the gym Taking an exercise class. Running. Cycling. Swimming. Weight training

I want to convince you that you are wrong if you think that you are unable to do exercise. The key is to change your understanding of exercise and to persuade you that you can do exercise – whoever you are.

Bad news / good news.

The bad news is you must get involved in some sort of exercise if you are going to achieve any weight loss and fitness level. You are genetically programmed to exercise and your body needs to be active is it is going to function in the way it has been designed to do so.

The good news is you do not need to become an Olympic athlete or 'hit the gym' to become fit and benefit from exercise. In fact, you already do exercise every day without realising it.

Yes, I am talking to anyone reading this book no matter how overweight or unfit that you think you are.

I will say this again for emphasis – anyone reading this book is already doing exercise every day of their life (unless completely confined to bed 24 hours a day).

The problem is you don't associate the things that you do every day with the fact that these are actually exercise.

The trick to help you lose weight and enjoy the benefits of a healthier lifestyle is to take the everyday activities you do (that is the true exercise you actually do without realising it) and *do them a bit more*!

This will make your heart beat faster and your lungs breathe more deeply. This will speed up your metabolism, which will burn more calories and fat.

You can benefit from using a wide variety of types of exercise programmes. Having said that, I would encourage you to maybe be ambitious in your exercise goals and think that perhaps you can achieve more than you think. I started off with a light exercise programme and gradually built up to the point where I have ran a half-marathon and qualified as a Fitness Instructor.

Am I saying that you should aim to run a half marathon? Certainly not! However, I surprised myself regarding the things that I was able to achieve. Perhaps you will be able to progress further than you ever imagined you could.

Don't worry about that at the moment – the important and key point is that you start to exercise and start to get the benefits now.

The key thing is taking it at a pace that you will actually sustain and keep going. It must become a natural part of your everyday life – just as eating habits must be re-educated, so must your exercise habits.

Time for an analogy: Think of when you started to learn to drive a car. Did you sit behind the steering wheel and start driving? Of course not! You followed a carefully planned series of lessons. As you became more skilful, your confidence increased, and you gradually developed the skills to drive the car competently and safely.

You pass your driving test when you can automatically do all that is required to drive the car without thinking about it. In other words, when you have developed all of the positive habits and skills required to drive a car at a subconscious level – it becomes second nature to you – a habit!

When you start an exercise programme, you are learning a new skill, and it takes time, just like learning to drive!

Exercise programmes

(In <u>addition</u> to *Exercise* – see page 113 - 114).

Exercise programmes on their own can be a bit like 'diets' for losing weight – they require willpower if you are going to stick to them. The problem is that most of us don't have the willpower to stick to fitness programmes – any more than we have the willpower to stick to the food and calorie restrictions of a diet programme.

Does this sound familiar?

The 1st of January arrives, and after the excesses of Christmas eating, you decide that you will set a New Year's resolution that you are going to lose weight and get fit. To achieve this, you start your diet and start an exercise programme.

This may involve joining a gym or renewing the membership you started last year but stopped using. Alternatively, you may opt to follow your new fitness programme at home and buy a fitness DVD and/or fitness equipment such as an exercise bike.

Let's fast forward a few weeks. You can't be bothered going to the gym anymore and the exercise DVD is in its box gathering dust, and the fitness equipment has become a clothes horse in the corner of the spare room or your bedroom.

Your good intentions to exercise will have fallen by the wayside! Why? The answer is simple – you are trying an 'exercise diet'. Unfortunately, an 'exercise diet' is just as useless as a food diet.

The parallels between a 'food diet' and 'exercise diet'.

	Initial Results	Long term results	Reason	Solution
Food Diet	Will have initial short-term results.	The results won't last. The weight will come back and more weight will be gained. You will feel bad about yourself.	Willpower doesn't work.	Re-educate eating habits. Follow: 'Three Point Plan'.
Exercise 'Diet' That is, exercise programmes, (*Level B or extra/add on activities*)	Will have initial short-term results.	The results won't last. The exercise programmes will stop. Your fitness levels will not improve. You will feel bad about yourself.	Willpower doesn't work.	Re-educate your thoughts about exercise. Remember the difference between '*exercise*' (Level A or ongoing everyday fitness) and Level B '*exercise programmes*'

Welcome to your new fitness programme!

Perhaps you could consider this to be day one of your new life of exercise. Remember, don't panic – think about all that I have said about exercise, relax and enjoy your new, positive, informed and enlightened attitude to exercise.

Your exercise lifestyle will be drawn from two levels:

Level A (*'exercise'*)	Your everyday daily activities	Walking, vacuuming and dusting your house, cutting the grass, etc.
Level B (*'exercise programmes'*)	An exercise programme that you enjoy.	Running, Zumba, cycling, aerobics, swimming, etc.

The 'Level A' *exercise* activities will be the foundation of your fitness.

The 'Level B' *exercise programmes* activities will be the *additional* things you can add onto the 'Level A' exercise activities.

This means that you will build your fitness upon the foundation of the natural way that you have been created and designed to do – by moving your body as is normal for your everyday life – only with a little more effort that results in your heart beating faster and your lungs breathing more deeply.

In practical terms, your will walk a little faster and a little farther each day; vacuum clean your carpet with a little more speed and effort; get out of a lift one floor down and walk up the remaining flight of stairs, etc.

'Level A' Exercise

(The foundation and main focus of your new fitness habit).

I will give some examples of *Level A* fitness activities. Here are just a few of the things you can do:

Walk a little bit faster:

When you are out walking, you could walk a little bit faster every so often. For example, you could alternate your walking speed between fast and slow, using lamp posts as your marker signal telling you when to change pace.

Walk a little bit farther:

Why not walk instead of getting the bus? Or, if it is too much to walk the full distance, why not get off the bus a few stops early and walk the rest of the way? You could even combine this with the technique stated above.

Or, if you live or work in a building requiring the use of a lift; perhaps you could get out of the lift one or two floors early and walk up the stairs to your destination floor.

Walk more often:

Can you walk somewhere instead of talking the car? Do you drive to the shop for a handful of items when you could walk?

If you only need a few items from the store, why not bring a backpack with you? When you walk home with the weight of the groceries in your backpack, you are adding another dimension to your exercise.

The examples stated above are only the tip of the iceberg' when it comes to finding ways to utilise the activities that you use every day to make you fitter.

Remember, this is the main focus and foundation of your fitness plan, and it will eventually become a natural part of your life – if you allow it to by keeping at it!

'Level B' Exercise *Programme*s

We are now going to think about supplementing the 'Level A' everyday exercise activities by doing a specific exercise programmes.

This is what we will be referring to as *'Level B' exercise programmes.* This is the harder bit – and it is the thing that has up to now, put you off exercise. The good news is that you have hopefully now changed your attitude to see the benefit of exercise.

This is how I recommend that you may go about establishing your 'Level B' fitness activities. You are an intelligent person and may want to find your own way and set out your own way of doing it.

Important points to remember before you begin any exercise programme.

Consult your doctor.

It is a good idea to check with your doctor before you start any new exercise programme, especially if you have not exercised for a while or have a medical history that may cause concern.

Know your limits.

Make sure that you follow exercise programmes appropriate to your current fitness levels, age and medical history. Expect to make progress as you get fitter; however, build up your fitness levels *gradually.*

Avoid exercise programmes which are likely to aggravate any medical conditions – there are plenty of exercise alternatives to choose from. If in doubt, discuss your concerns with a suitably qualified Fitness Instructor or Personal Trainer. Your local leisure centre is a good place to start.

Listen to your body.

Do not continue to exercise through pain, fatigue, breathlessness or dizziness. If you experience any of these symptoms, your body is communicating to you that it has had enough or is being hurt in some way. You must STOP immediately.

Patience is the key!

Remember; do not try to too much too soon. It is important to build up your fitness gradually. Remember the earlier analogy of learning to drive a car?

Here are some practical steps to help you plan and develop your *Level B exercise programme.*

Step 1

Decide <u>*what*</u> activities you would like to do.

It is important to do an exercise activity that you will enjoy and actually keep doing in the long term.

For example, are you going to:

Take up running?
Join a gym?
Take some fitness classes?
Take up swimming?
Buy a fitness DVD?
Buy some home gym equipment?
Buy a bike?

I will strike a note of caution here!

Please do not let past negative experiences of certain activities put you off being open-minded about the possibilities on offer.

This is a new start and it is important to be open-minded, because you might surprise yourself! I know that I surprised myself by the fitness activities I enjoy and benefitted from.

Step 2

Decide <u>*how*</u> you are going to do the exercise programme.

In other words, make a plan of the exercise programmes that you are going to do (in addition to your 'Level A' everyday fitness activities programme).

It is important to think about this carefully as you need to make sure that you get the most out of your exercise programme.

Step 3

Decide <u>when</u> you are going to do the exercise programme.

You will need to decide:

- How often you are going to do your exercise programme.
- How long you are going to spend doing the exercise programme
- What time of day you are going to do your exercise programme.

We will now look at these points in more detail.

How often are you going to do your new exercise programme?

Once you have decided which exercise programme you are going to do, it is vital to make sure that you are realistic about how long you are going to perform the exercise, and the length and intensity of each session.

Here are some important things to think about:

Set realistic targets for yourself.

Here are two key things for you to remember:

- Do not spend too long exercising in one session.
- Do not exercise the same muscle groups too often in one week without leaving at least a day in between to allow the muscles to recover.

It is important to let the body get ready for exercise gradually, especially if you have not been involved in exercise for a while. This is an important principle of Nature.

If you try too much too soon you risk injury and discouragement, which may result in giving up. Your muscles and nervous system need to get used to the extra workload being placed on them by the requirements of the exercise programme.

Every time you exercise, a whole series of complicated actions take place in your body as it adjusts to the extra demands being placed on it by the force of the exercise.

We all have a fitness level, and when our body reaches that fitness level, it will inform the brain that it has hit maximum level and we will be warned to stop by our body. If we ignore that warning signal to stop, we can over-strain the body and cause injury.

Every time we exercise, we must challenge the systems in our body and stretch them to a certain point and then stop. The next time we exercise, the body will have been conditioned to cope with a little bit more pressure, and be able to deal with the new level of overload more efficiently.

This is how you get fitter!

Also, the body will only respond positively to, and benefit from, an exercise session for so long. After a while, the body will reach the limit of what it can get from the exercise. The technical term for this is 'Plateau'.

Once your body hits the limit (plateau), the exercise actually stops being effective. This means that you are actually wasting your time by continuing with the workout as your body has got all it is going to get out of the exercise.

In fact, it will become counter-productive and start to harm your body. Exercising too long can lead to injury and other problems

Please remember, if you can only manage four or five minutes, then you should stick to doing the activity for this length of time.

If you try to push yourself beyond the limits of your current fitness level, you will hurt yourself and become discouraged.

Three minutes at the start of your exercise programme will become four minutes, which will become five minutes (and so on) as your fitness levels *gradually* improve.

Be patient as less is more!

The importance of Rest

One of the most common mistake made by people when they begin an exercise programme, is to think that the more often they perform a certain exercise, the fitter they will become.

In fact, the opposite is true – less is actually more!

It is not the exercise that gets us fit, it is the ***recovery*** that happens during the 24 – 48 hour period *after* the exercise has been performed that we get fit.

Let me explain:

Every time you perform an exercise activity, small tears occur in your muscles. These tears are subsequently repaired by our body, and the repairs make the muscle stronger. If we exercise that muscle before the small tears in the muscle have been repaired, the tears from the previous session will still not be fully repaired.

Therefore, the muscle fibres will be torn again too soon, and they will not become stronger. This means that you will not get the full fitness benefit from your workout.

By rest, I don't mean *inactivity*. Rest in this context means not using the same muscle group again for 48 hours. For example, if you run on Monday, do not run again until Wednesday. On the Tuesday in-between, you should do a different type of exercise which will focus on different muscle groups. For example, exercise your upper body in order to give your legs and knees time to repair, recover and become fitter.

Remember, less is more!

What time of day will you exercise?

Are you a lark or an owl?

In other words, are you a natural morning person who tends to function best in the morning (a lark)? Or, are you a person who naturally likes to 'burn the midnight oil' and functions best late in the evening (an owl)?

A lot of recent research has strongly suggested that Nature has decided whether we are natural morning or evening people. This has been determined by our genes.

Does our natural inclination to being either a lark or owl have any bearing on the time of day we should perform our exercise programmes?

The answer appears to be 'yes'.

It appears that some people get more benefit from exercising in the evening, and in contrast, other people will benefit most from exercising in the morning – depending on whether you have been genetically programmed to be a lark or an owl.

The time of day that we naturally favour for the maximum exercise benefits is due to a natural body rhythm called the *circadian rhythm.*

What is the circadian rhythm?

The circadian rhythm is more commonly referred to as our 'body clock'.

Our own unique circadian rhythm is a 24-hour cycle that controls all of the physical and behavioural processes and changes that happens in our body. It controls things such as our body temperature, heart rate, blood pressure, chemical and hormone levels, cell regeneration, sleep patterns, etc.

The circadian rhythm will affect each of us differently, therefore, it is essential to understand how *your* body clock is programmed.

Early morning exercise.

<u>Warning</u>: early morning may be the worst time of day for *you* to perform exercise!

There are a lot of early morning exercise classes in some of the gyms and leisure centres at the moment. Also, there are a lot of people who advocate getting up early and performing some sort of exercise before they go to work.

However; are early morning exercise programmes right and safe for *you*?

Remember, we each have this unique daily body rhythm (circadian rhythm) that controls every aspect of how our body functions.

It is strongly suggested by current scientific research that early morning is the worst time for *some* people to engage in exercise programmes and activities.

The reason for this is because the state of the body systems of many people has not been 'set' by the body clock (circadian rhythm) to the best and safest level for exercise in the morning.

When we wake up in the morning, we begin the process of getting into gear for the day ahead. Our systems start to warm up.

Upon awakening, our blood is usually thicker, our blood vessels are usually more rigid and our blood pressure will usually take time to adjust to the demands of the day ahead. Also, our muscles are usually tighter and require time to loosen. In fact, some scientists have called this time of day the 'heart attack danger zone'.

In light of all this, early morning exercise can be a very bad time of day for *you* to perform an exercise programme because your system may not warm up quickly enough for your body to fully benefit from the exercise programme you are following. It can also be counter-productive as you may actually hurt yourself.

Therefore, it may be better for *you* to exercise later in the day.

Interestingly, current scientific research is suggesting that the principle of the unsuitability of early morning exercise my also apply to some top professional and elite sportsmen and women.

The research suggests that the traditional early morning training for professional sports people may actually be counter-productive, and some may actually improve their performance by moving their training to later in the day, depending on the individual body clock. It has been suggested that the success of Spanish football teams may be due to their culture of starting later – an interesting thought!

On the other hand, it may well be that *you* are a morning person and early morning exercise programmes suit *you*. The key is making sure that you follow your exercise programmes at a time that suits your circadian rhythm!

Start your (Level B) exercise programme.

There are many exercise programmes for you to choose from, and it is important to choose a programme that you will enjoy and stick with.

Remember, it is important have an open mind when you are deciding which exercise programme you are choosing, and don't let past negative experiences put you off.

There are too many programmes out there for me to list in this book. You can contact your local gym or leisure centre to find out the programmes on offer. Also, there are many exercise programmes available on DVD or the internet.

Some of these programmes are very good and beneficial – I use some of them myself. However, the problem with a DVD or the internet is that quality assurance cannot be guaranteed as anyone can make a video and post it online. Make sure the video or DVD is presented by a reputable organisation and suitably qualified individuals.

I offer you my best wishes as you now begin your journey to your new level of fitness. You will be glad you did as it will improve the quality of your life.

Chapter 17

Let's think food - First change *how* you eat, then change *what* you eat

Let's get real about eating.

You live in the real world – not an academic, analytical, 100% scientifically accurate world where you analyse all of the ingredients contained in all of the food you eat to make sure that you are putting the perfect food types into your body.

We are too busy getting on with our life and daily activities to have the time or inclination to measure fat content, count calories or work out all of the scientific data regarding the foods we buy every time we go shopping. Furthermore, we have settled into a routine and habit of eating the type of food items with which we fill our fridge and cupboards.

Think about your shopping habits for a moment. You will go to the supermarket, collect your trolley and begin the 'battle of the shopping trip'. I call it a battle because you will be entering the world of the modern retailer, and this is a world of hassle and stress. Consider some of the things that you will experience is you battle through the supermarket aisles:

- Your own tiredness as you have had a long hard day at work or looking after your family.

- Your own financial situation - the amount you have to spend on your food and sticking to your household budget.

- Other shoppers who suddenly stop in front of you, suddenly change direction or push their trolley at great speed through the store and don't give way or slow down.

- People who block the entire section of shelf you want with their trolley and won't move, because they are having difficulty deciding which brand to choose.

- You are walking towards the checkout with a few items in your basket; however, another shopper with a trolley full of items deliberately runs and beats you to the queue.

- The atmosphere created by the supermarket. All supermarkets are deliberately designed to keep you in a constant state of sensory discomfort and overload. This results in you spending more money in the store. You also have to endure screaming children and annoying background music, etc.

- Confusing price labels. Is the 'buy one get one free' good value? Is the supermarket brand really better value than the more expensive leading brand?

Realistically, once you factor all of the above into your shopping trip, the last thing you will want to do is stand

and count the calories and agonise over the fat and salt content contained in the food that you buy.

Thankfully, it is not necessary to change your shopping habits all at once during the first phase of your weight loss journey.

Once you have re-educated your eating habits by focussing on *how* you should eat, you can then move onto *what* you should eat. As you gradually change your *eating habits*, you will find that you will find it easier to change your *shopping habits* and move to eating healthier food items. You will also be able to keep eating many of the foods you currently eat and enjoy.

Remember, the key to permanent weight loss and weight management is to follow the following practices, in the following order of priority:

Replace old *faulty* eating habits by establishing *good* eating habits by following the 'Three Point Plan'.

Eat a good, sensible, well balanced intake of food that will enable you to be the healthiest version of yourself.

In other words:

First, we must change: *How* we eat!

Then, we change: *What* we eat!

The key to this weight loss programme is that at the beginning, you *do not dramatically change what you eat all at once – no food is banned or prohibited at the start of your weight loss journey.*

Once you have established your new eating habits, you can start thinking about the foods you should and shouldn't eat. By following the approach outlined in this book, you will find it easier to gradually replace some of the unhealthy food types (and portions) with healthier options. It will eventually become natural and second nature to you – *if* you follow the programme. You don't rely on willpower, which doesn't work anyway. The more you try to cut out and ban a certain food, the more you will want it.

Question: Surely we should only try to put good and healthy food into body from the start of our weight loss programme?

Answer: Yes, in an ideal world you should; however, we don't live in an ideal world. Realistically, you are not going to suddenly change your shopping and eating habits. To do this requires willpower - something most of us don't have in sufficient strength to sustain a sudden change of eating and shopping behaviour. You will change for a while and then fall back into your old ways.

Explanation: Trying to suddenly change your food intake will result in your body going into 'famine mode' as you are basically *'going on a diet'*. Remember, diets don't work and you must gradually replace your bad eating habits with good eating habits by following a natural weight loss programme, such as the one outlined in this book.

Question: *Surely this means that we will continue to eat things that are bad for us – the things that make us overweight and unhealthy?*

Answer: Yes, *at first* we will continue to put the unhealthy things into or body – *for a while!* However, we must look at the bigger picture.

Explanation: As the old saying puts it, *'sometimes you need to lose the battle in order to win the war'*. Another old saying tells us that, *'sometimes it needs to get worse before it gets better'*. The key to permanent weight loss is re-educating our eating habits. It took time for us to develop the old bad eating habits; therefore, logic tells us that it will take time to gradually replace these with the good, natural eating habits required to maintain a healthy weight.

At the beginning of the programme, we will inevitably put into our bodies things that we shouldn't. However, we will make up for this later once we have established our new natural eating habits.

Our body is wonderfully designed and created and Nature has programmed it to deal with the waste and rubbish, and still be very healthy and fit - as long as the rubbish is the *lesser* amount and not the greater.

I really cannot be bothered counting calories or going through some of the technical details regarding the contents of all of the food I eat. The good news is we don't need to.

What foods can we eat?

We know that we need certain key nutrients to keep our body alive and healthy. However, we don't eat nutrients and flavours; rather, we eat *food* which *contains* the *nutrients and flavours* we both *need* and *like.*

How do we know if we are eating the right amount of fibre, sugar, carbohydrates, protein, etc?

You could try to count every gram and percentages contained in each food item, and use a calculator to work out if you are eating the right amount of each ingredient and nutrient.

If you do decide to take this approach – I wish you luck, as I know that I can't be bothered to live like this, and I know that many other people won't be able to either. I found that this approach was unrealistic, unhelpful and unnecessary. Quite frankly, it is 'over-egging the pudding' if you pardon the pun!

Question: '*Does this mean that we don't need to take time to think about the calories, fat content, ingredients and macronutrients in our food?*'

Answer: No, we need to have an *awareness* of the balance of the ingredients and nutrients contained in our food; however, we can achieve an appropriate balance of the things we need to eat healthily by following a few simple guidelines:

- Follow the principles of the 'Three Point Plan'.
- Have a basic awareness of the types of nutrients your body requires to maintain an appropriate weight and remain healthy.
- Make sure that you try eat a balanced mixture of food items taken from the following food groups listed in the table below:

1	Bread, rice, potatoes, pasta, variety of other starchy foods
2	Fruit & vegetables
3	Milk & dairy foods
4	Meat, fish, eggs, beans plus protein from other non-dairy sources
5	Fat (as appropriate)
6	Sugar (in limited amounts)
7	Fluids, including lots of water in addition to tea and coffee, etc

It is *how* we eat, the *amount* we eat and the *combination* of the good and bad nutrients in the food that will determine the size of our waistline and the quality of our fitness and health.

Jargon Alert:

I will give a brief explanation of the key terms and concepts you will come across when exploring what we should and should not eat. I will explain terms such as cholesterol, protein, carbohydrates, and different types of fats, etc.

We should be aiming to eat a food intake in which has a balance of the following *essential* nutrients (or '*Macronutrients*' to use the technical term).

	Examples	Function
Carbohydrates	Rice, pasta, potatoes, bread, cereals, grains, etc.	Energy production
Fats	Dairy products, fish, nuts, seeds, oils (olive oil, etc)	Energy production and insulation.
Proteins	Meat, dairy products, nuts, beans, eggs, chicken	Repair and growth of body tissue

Carbohydrates: Provides energy for the body and is broken down into glucose, which provides fuel that is required to be used by all of the tissues in our body.

Carbohydrates come in two forms:

- *Simple carbohydrates* – sugars which naturally occur and are found in milk and fruit.
- *Complex carbohydrates* - starches found in plants, such as grains, seeds, potatoes and other root vegetables.

Protein: This is the building material that our body requires for both repair and growth of all the tissues in our body. Protein can also be broken down by our body and used as energy during long periods of activity.

Fat: It is essential for our health and well-being that we put fat into our body. It only becomes a problem when we eat *too much* and the *wrong type* of fat. Fat is stored and used as a fuel supply for our body, and also as insulation to help our body regulate and prevent heat loss.

Here is a list of how fat contributes to some of the key functions in our body:

- Providing fuel for energy
- Providing insulation for our body
- Maintaining cells

- Manufacturing hormones
- Transporting fat-soluble vitamins
- Maintaining brain function

We store two types of fat.

The body stores fat in two different ways – *subcutaneous* fat and *visceral* fat. It is very important that we understand the difference between these different types of fat and the impact they can have on our health and well-being.

Subcutaneous fat:

This is the fat that we store on our body just under the skin. We recognise this type of fat because we can feel (or 'pinch') it under the skin.

Visceral fat:

Visceral fat is also known as 'abdominal fat' or 'active fat' because it is stored in the abdomen and, more seriously, around the internal organs.

Visceral fat is more dangerous to our health than subcutaneous fat, and is associated with many serious health problems and conditions such as type 2 diabetes, high blood pressure and cardiovascular disease, etc. We cannot feel visceral fat as it is too deeply stored within our body.

Types of fat in our food.

There are basically four main types of fat to be found in our food, and these types of fat are usually classified as *'good fat'* or *'bad fat'*.

- Monounsaturated fat.
- Polyunsaturated fat.
- Saturated fat.
- Trans-fats.

The various types of fat perform different roles within our body, and will have very different effects on our health – either for good or bad! These fat types are divided into 'good' and 'bad' as follows:

Good fat	Monounsaturat ed fat	This fat is to be found in food types such as nuts, avocado, olives and olive oil.
Good fat	Polyunsaturated fat.	Come in two types, omega 3 and Omega 6. This fat is found in sunflower oil, corn, nuts, fish, vegetable oil, etc.
'Bad' fat	Saturated fat*	This fat comes mostly from animals such as red meat, poultry and full fat dairy products.
Very bad fat (Some call this 'Killer' fat).	Trans-fats.	This fat is man-made from oils using a process called 'partial hydrogenation'. It is found in deep-fried food, some take-away meals, some baked goods such as pies, sausage rolls, pastries, cakes, biscuits and buns. Trans-fats are not found in Nature!

*Some current research is questioning if 'saturated fat' in some foods (e.g. dairy products), in moderation, is as 'bad' for our health as previously thought. I look into this further in the next chapter.

Question: does this mean that we should not eat any food with the 'bad' fat?

Answer: In a perfect world it would, but we don't live in a perfect world. No food is banned if we are following this natural weight loss programme and we can eat 'bad' things within reason.

The key word is *balance!*

Cholesterol: This is a fatty substance which is vital for the body to function normally. The technical term for cholesterol is lipid. There are two types of lipids: 'Bad' and 'good'.

- HDL (High Density Lipoprotein). This is 'good' cholesterol. This goes back to the liver where it is broken down or eliminated from the body as a waste product.
- LDL (Low Density Lipoprotein). This is 'bad' cholesterol. We do need this; however, if we eat too much of this type, it can build up on the artery walls leading to disease.

It is recommended that you get your cholesterol checked regularly by means of a simple blood test by your family doctor.

Chapter 18

These are a few of my favourite things

Unlike many 'diet books', I am not going to give you a list of the foods you should avoid while losing weight. Instead, I am going to discuss some of the popular foods many diet books say you should avoid, and show that you may be still able to eat these 'banned' items while re-educating your eating habits to achieve permanent weight loss.

I am not going to write about every food – just some of my favourites.

Butter, margarine and other low fat spreads.

Butter

Butter has been a favorite spread of choice for many people for generations. I remember from my childhood eating my hot toast dripping with lovely creamy butter – my mouth is watering now as I think back. In those days, however, there was not the same consciousness about the health or fat issues. We ate butter and thought nothing of it. Now there is great alarm among the health conscious.

Butter is made with milk or cream by being churned in large purpose-built vats. The key fact from the point of view of our discussion is the amount of fat contained in butter.

Question: Do we need to stop eating butter because of the fat?

The fear of fat in our diets and the effect it can have on our bodies (excess weight and heart disease) is the main driving force behind the move by many people away from butter. I was one of them, but I am not quite so sure now.

It is now suggested by some current research that butter may actually be acceptable and perhaps even better for us than the margarines and low fat spreads which have replaced butter in many households.

A senior medical doctor (a consultant cardiologist) on a TV morning news programme said that he eats butter, as do many of his medical colleagues, and recommends that everyone else should eat it.

Also, one of my relatives was discussing weight management and healthy eating with her family doctor. Her doctor said that she ate only butter and avoided margarine and spreads. Furthermore, the doctor recommends that her patients do the same. This view is also reflected in many examples of current literature and online articles.

Current research is questioning the commonly held opinion that the fat (especially saturated fat) in butter, eggs, cheese, full-fat milk, etc, is as harmful to our health as previously thought (especially concerning heart disease).

The current understanding of the way we digest saturated fat has been cast into doubt. Put simply, although eating butter (and other dairy products such as cheese) is putting saturated fat into our digestive system, it is suggested that a large proportion of the fat passes through our system and out of our body - eliminated in our waste when we go to the toilet.

Therefore, not as much fat is absorbed into our body. Thus it may not have the negative effect on our waistline or cholesterol as researchers once believed.

Butter v Low Fat Spreads/Margarine

One of the positive things we can say about butter is it is produced with the use of *minimal processing* and is a *natural food* made from the natural products from milk fat alone. This fat is, of course, taken from the pure and natural substance of milk.

Spreads have become very popular because they are 'Low Fat' alternatives to butter. In contrast to butter, these spreads are produced by means of *heavy processing*, and contain many *artificial additives, chemicals, colourings, preservatives* and a mixture of unsaturated oils such as olive oil, sunflower oil and rapeseed oil.

This does not mean that these products are necessarily bad and to be avoided; however, it does mean that we need to take the time to actually look at the benefits of these products compared to butter when we are deciding what we should spread on our toast and sandwiches.

Which should I use - butter or low fat spreads?

I really wish that I could give you a definitive answer; however, here is a summary of some of the key positives and negatives associated with each product. You are an intelligent person and you must look at the various spreads available and decide whether butter or low fat spreads fits best into your healthy lifestyle. Remember, let the waistband of your trousers or skirt and cholesterol level be your guide – the key word is *balance*!

Summary of the positives and negatives associated with butter and margarine/spreads:

Butter	
Positives	Negatives
Is made from natural ingredients. Is made using natural processes (churning).	Has a high level of saturated fat. Current research is now suggesting that saturated fat in moderation may not be as bad for us as previously thought. We need fat and the fat content may be ok if it is balanced within the limits of our total fat intake.

Margarine / Spreads	
Positives	Negatives
Most of these spreads have low saturated fat.	These spreads are made from 'man made' processes. They contain more 'trans-fats' which according to many researchers, are more of a risk to health than saturated fat. They have additives and chemicals in them. Are chemicals more potentially harmful in the long term to our health than the 'natural' fat in butter?

Hedge your bets

Spreads are available which are attempting to be the '*best of both worlds*' between butter and low fat spreads. Maybe this is the answer. The manufacturers claim that this product has been naturally produced by using naturally low fat buttermilk, which has been 'skimmed' from the churn. It is said to have the buttery taste; however, it is supposed to contain half the saturated fat of butter and only natural flavour and colour. Significantly, it is claimed that it doesn't contain any hydrogenated fats and isn't manufactured by means of heavy man-made processing.

I have to take these claims at face value and trust that the powers that be have protected us from any false claims.

This type of product is halfway between full butter and low fat spreads. Yes, it probably is sitting on the fence to a certain extent to use this possible 'best of both worlds' product. However, sitting on the fence is sitting in the middle, which possibly could be interpreted as another way of finding the 'balance'.

Ultimately you '*pay your money and make your choice*'!

Milk

I remember as a child waking up each morning to a distinctive sound of the clinking of bottles and sound of the electric engine of a funny little vehicle - the milk float of our local milkman doing his rounds. I also remember in my early years at primary school getting my little bottle of milk every morning break-time, until the government put an end to this.

Sadly, the sight of a milkman is quite rare these days as only a lucky few still have a local milkman service. Most of us now get our milk from the supermarket or other local shops.

The method of delivery has changed, but the amount of milk we drink has changed little. The official statistics show that people in the UK drink over five billion litres of milk per year.

Most of us buy milk without thinking as a part of our daily or weekly shopping. It is one of those things that most of us make sure that we don't run out of. How many times do we 'nip to the shop' for some milk?

Milk is a masterpiece of Nature and is packed with goodness and many fantastic ingredients. For example, a single glass of milk contains the following things which are vital to the good health of our body:

- Calcium (equivalent level to 41 Bananas)
- Protein
- Carbohydrate
- Vitamins (A, B, C, etc.)
- Iodine
- Iron
- Magnesium
- Potassium
- Fluoride
- Fat (remember, our body needs the appropriate amount and type of fat).

Some people experience difficulty with milk; however, sometimes it is certain elements within milk such as *lactose* and *casein* that are the source of difficulty.

Lactose free milk is available and you may be able to enjoy the great benefits of milk via one of these modified products.

An interesting benefit of milk

One benefit of milk that you may not know about – it is a good *recovery drink*!

It is good to drink milk after vigorous activity because it can help our muscles recover more quickly. Vigorous activity includes exercise, working hard in the garden, painting and decorating etc.

I know from my studies to become a Fitness Instructor that vigorous activity and exercise puts stress on our muscles and that it will typically take 48 hours for them to recover. One of the effects of activity is the release of chemicals into our blood called *creatine kinase* and *myoglobin*. The rates at which these settle and are absorbed by our blood indicate how quickly our muscles recover.

Milk can contribute to the lowering of these chemicals and help to promote faster muscle recovery because it contains <u>both</u> *carbohydrates* and *protein*. Carbohydrates help to *reduce the breakdown* of muscle tissue after exercise and protein actually *rebuilds* the muscle tissue.

This two-fold *reactive* and *proactive* effect restores the muscle tissue damage much more quickly than sports recovery drinks, which only have the one element of reduction of muscle damage (carbohydrate).

This combination of protein and carbohydrate is found in equal measure in skimmed, semi-skimmed and full-fat milk.

Skimmed, semi-skimmed of full-fat milk.

What type of milk should we use if we want to achieve and maintain a healthy weight?

The answer is – it depends! Sorry that I don't have a definitive answer. You need to decide how much fat you think you should be taking. I drink Semi-skimmed because it is a balance and compromise between skimmed milk (which many people find too 'thin' and can't acquire the taste for) and full fat milk (which many think contains unhelpful levels of fat). Again, please look into the alternatives and use your common sense to make your decision.

Cheese

I love cheese, and I am not alone! According to a recent survey, 65% of adults in the UK say that cheese is one of their favourite food items. In addition to being delicious, cheese is packed with a host of nutrients such as calcium, protein, zinc, vitamins, etc. Cheese is very versatile and comes in a variety of types, flavours and textures, and can be used in a wide variety of ways.

What about the fat in cheese?

Many points discussed regarding fat in butter also apply to cheese so I won't repeat them. Cheese is a fantastic food we can eat and enjoy. Balance is the key. Let the waistband of your trousers or skirt and your cholesterol level be your guide as to whether you are eating too much.

Low fat varieties of cheese are also available.

Eggs

I can remember from my childhood an old TV advertisement which said *'I like eggs, good for you and helps build muscle'*. Interesting claims, but are they true?

Also, on the internet I came across another superb TV advertisement from the 1970s featuring the late great football legend George Best. In this advert engages in conversation with a schoolboy who asks him for his autograph. George says he didn't play well in a recent match because he didn't have his usual egg for breakfast.

Obviously George was paid to take part in this advertisement; however, is there something in what he said about eating an egg to help our performance during the day?

The benefits of eggs

Eggs are a very nutrient-dense food item containing many fantastic ingredients which are very beneficial to our health. Protein, vitamins (A, B, B12, D), iron, zinc are a few of the major nutrients in eggs.

Question: Surely eggs are not good for us because they are full of fat and can raise our cholesterol?

Eggs have received a very bad press recently with the 'eggs are high in fat and cholesterol' statement being quoted in a forceful way. This has now found its way strongly into the public consciousness and has put a lot of people off eating eggs.

They do contain fat; however, many of the points discussed regarding the fat in butter also apply to eggs. Most heart and health organisations are questioning and amending their recommendations regarding egg consumption, as current scientific opinion is suggesting that the fat in eggs may not have as significant an effect on blood cholesterol as was previously thought.

In common with butter, milk and other dairy products, it is also suggested by current research that not as much of the fat is absorbed into our digestive system as was previously thought.

The key word is *balance!*

Sandwiches

What are you going to eat for your lunch? If this were a diet book, you might be told to ditch sandwiches in favour of a list containing a variety of 'diet foods'. Let's get real! First of all, this is not a diet book. You are not going to stop eating sandwiches, and the good news is you don't need to cut them out of your natural healthy eating habits.

People love sandwiches, and this is borne out by the fact that over 2 billion pre-prepared sandwiches are sold in various retail outlets every year in the UK alone. On top of this figure, we have no way of knowing the exact amount of sandwiches prepared at home for packed lunches for school and work.

What are the best fillings to put into our sandwiches to help us manage our weight?

We should go for fillings which keep us *fuller-for-longer* to stop us from being tempted to snack in mid-afternoon. One of the best ways to achieve this is to try to make sure that our sandwiches have plenty of *protein,* which is broken down a slower rate in our stomach and will make us feel full.

Here are a few examples of sandwich fillings which are full of protein and will help to keep you fuller for longer and stop you from having the mid-afternoon nibbles:

Chicken is a great option and possible the best option as it absolutely packed with protein.

Cheese and tomato is another good option. You can opt for a low fat variety of cheese if you are concerned about fat content.

Egg and cress is another good option.

Please remember that *gluten free bread* can be used by those with a problem in this area.

Soup

Soup can actually help us eat less and provide us with lots of nutritional goodness.

How can eating soup help me to manage my weight?

First, choose the soup that will provide you with the most health benefits and keep you *fuller for longer*. It is better to choose soups with ingredients such as chunky vegetables. You should avoid creamy soups.

Research has shown us that after we eat the soup with the best ingredients (chunky vegetables, etc), a large amount stays in and stretches our stomach and is digested slowly. This sends the signal that we are full and should stop eating.

Soup as a starter.

We can leave food on the plate at home if we follow the principle of *stop eating when full*; however, at certain social situations it may offend your host if you leave food on your plate.

It is fine to modify *the 'Three Point plan'* at special times, such as when you go out for a meal or attend a special function. However, a good trick you can use to help you not to overeat is to take a healthy soup as a starter. This will leave less room in your stomach and can help ensure that you go for smaller portions from the main course menu.

Nuts

Not everyone can take nuts as some people suffer from nut allergy. If you can take them, nuts really are another masterpiece of Nature. They really are a fantastic option if you fancy a snack, and are a much better choice than crisps/potato chips or popcorn, etc.

Why are nuts so good for us?

There are many different types of nuts out there and they all have benefits. Nuts are packed with nutrients such as protein, fibre, calcium, vitamins, riboflavin, and niacin to mention but a few. It is also suggested by some research that eating nuts, such as almonds, may actually help the body fight off viral infections such as the common cold and flu. The skin of the almond contains chemicals which help white blood cells to deal with these viruses. This helps to prevent them from spreading in the body.

Also, some recent research has suggested that eating nuts five times a week could possibly contribute to reducing the risk of a heart attack.

Objection,

Perhaps you are thinking that nuts are not such a good healthy option because they *'contain high levels of fat'*

You are correct, nuts are full of fat; however, the really great news is that they have large amounts of the so called 'good fat' – the type of fat that lowers cholesterol, and is currently thought of as being good for our health in general.

Furthermore, research has shown us that when we eat nuts, a high amount of the fat contained in nuts actually passes through our digestive process and out of our system when we pass our waste into the toilet. This means that a lot of the fat in the nuts passes through our system without being absorbed into our body.

Eating whole nuts will provide us with the greatest benefit. Nut products such as peanut butter or finely chopped nuts are also beneficial, but the nutrients are affected by the preparation processes.

Beans

I am referring primarily to 'Baked Beans'.

Beans are associated with the diet of students as they are learning to survive at university, or single people who can't be bothered to cook a full meal when they come home from work. We also think of beans as being part of kids' meal option at restaurants. However, it you think that beans are just for students or children, then you need to think again!

Why are beans so good for us?

They contain many great things that our body requires to remain healthy. Here is a list of some of the main healthy things found in beans:

Protein: The 'building blocks' of our body - important for growth, maintenance and repair (beans on 2 slices of wholemeal toast has the same level of protein as a sirloin steak – at a fraction of the cost).

Amino acids: Beans provide the body with a wide range of amino acids, which we really cannot do without.

Insoluble Fibre: The shell of the beans contains insoluble fibre which serves to help keep our digestive system healthy.

Soluble Fibre: The inside of the bean contains soluble fibre which helps to lower cholesterol, control blood sugar levels and can help feel fuller for longer.

Please don't overlook beans or underestimate their value in terms of how good they are for you. Remember, you can make yourself a very good and healthy meal very easily and quickly, with little cost.

Chocolate

What? Chocolate in a weight loss and fitness book! Have I taken leave of my senses?

When I was overweight I was shocked when I monitored the amount of chocolate I ate in a single day – sometimes three or four chocolate bars plus lots of chocolate biscuits. Many people, and I was one of them, would say that they are 'addicted' to chocolate – a 'chocoholic'. I would say that I had 'withdrawal symptoms' if I didn't get my 'fix' of chocolate.

Chocolate is probably the food that most people 'who go on a diet' struggle the most to 'cut out' in order to lose weight. The great news is we are not on a diet and no food is banned. I still eat chocolate, but the key word is *occasionally* - balance is the key!

Question: Is chocolate addictive in the same way as alcohol or nicotine?

Answer: Not really! We eat chocolate because we *really like the taste* and it brings us *pleasure.*

It is suggested by the researchers that eating chocolate stimulates key areas of the brain and brings pleasure. It may stimulate the same parts of the brain associated with addiction, but this is not the same as having a physical addiction.

In some ways I was disappointed that I wasn't really addicted to chocolate, as this would have given me an excuse to over-indulge and not take any blame or responsibility, as it was my brain forcing me to get a fix to satisfy my addiction – just like smokers need a cigarette to get their nicotine fix.

We have developed a *habit* of eating chocolate because we *love* the taste. This means that we can re-educate ourselves to develop a new chocolate eating habit.

Therefore, the really good news is we do not need to give up chocolate completely. I always treat myself to chocolate at the weekends.

What about craving? Yes, occasionally I crave chocolate; however, thanks to my re-educated eating habits, I can deal with the cravings by following the techniques outlined in the *'Cravings – the enemy of weight loss'* chapter of this book.

Fantastic news - Chocolate is good for you!

The media is currently highlighting the recent research stating that we should eat chocolate for the benefit of our health – in *moderation*!

The health benefits of chocolate

Research suggests that eating chocolate can actually be good for you as it possesses a number of natural ingredients that are beneficial for our health. These ingredients are found in both milk chocolate and dark chocolate; however, the extra fat and sugar in the milk variety makes it a less healthy option than the dark chocolate.

Some examples of how eating chocolate may be good for you:

The Heart – It may help to prevent arteriosclerosis (hardening of the arteries) and prevent blood clots because it improves blood flow. It may also help to lower blood pressure.

The Brain – It may contribute to improved blood flow to the brain, which may help to reduce the risk of stroke and also improve concentration and cognitive function.

Your mood - It may also help to make you feel happier. The chemicals in the chocolate encourage your brain to release *endorphins* – the 'feel good' chemical and *phenylethylamine*, the 'fall in love' chemical that is released when you experience the 'high' in the early stages of falling in love!

Your general health – chocolate contains vitamins and minerals, such as iron, etc. Also, just like tea, chocolate contains antioxidants, albeit in much smaller amounts.

Dark chocolate may contain a chemical that may help to strengthen the enamel on our teeth and also help control blood sugar level thus helping to protect against diabetes.

If you can cope with it, dark chocolate is a healthier option and could be helpful to our waistline as it is an acquired taste. It is not as easy to eat in large quantities because it doesn't taste as good as milk chocolate which has more sugar and fat mixed into it. Dark chocolate does contain caffeine, but much less than tea & coffee. It also contains sugar, but much less than milk chocolate.

A few squares from a bar of dark chocolate can be a good snack!

Desserts

Can we really enjoy dessert and still manage our weight?

Yes, you can enjoy the occasional dessert and still control your weight. We are not following a ‘diet’ with all of the associated restrictions.

Remember, the Hedonic appetite pathway (eating for pleasure)? We have been created to eat to live and to enjoy eating - this is Nature’s way: however, desserts should only be taken *occasionally* and ‘be our servant, not our master’.

Here are some practical tips to help you enjoy desserts without piling on the pounds:

- Don’t eat a dessert after every meal – only as a weekend treat or on special occasions.

- Eat slowly and make each mouthful last as long as possible.

- Stop when you are full in your *stomach* – not your *head*!

Chapter 19

Breakfast - the most important meal of the day

You have probably heard it said that breakfast is the most important meal of the day. My experience has led me to the conclusion that this statement is true. In fact, I am now firmly convinced that you will find it more difficult to lose weight on a permanent basis if you do not establish the good habit of starting your day by eating breakfast.

A good breakfast will have the positive ingredients and properties that will keep you feeling 'fuller-for-longer' and release energy on a slow and steady basis. A fried breakfast every day is not a really good breakfast; however, if you are following this proven-by-experience natural way of weight management, you can have a fried breakfast occasionally.

Objection: Some people say: *'I just cannot eat breakfast – I will be sick if I do'*

I used to say that I couldn't eat breakfast; however, this was due to *conditioning* and *habit*. You need to re-educate your eating habits to include eating breakfast or you will find it more difficult to lose weight and keep it off.

Why does eating a good breakfast help us keep off the pounds?

If you get up and rush out of the house without eating any breakfast you are not giving any fuel to your body. It is important to eat a good breakfast because it will fill you up and you will not feel hungry again until lunchtime.

This will help you to only *eat when truly hungry in your stomach ('tummy hungry')*, resulting in avoiding eating snacks at mid-morning tea-break. I was amazed by the amount of food that I ate at morning tea-break. I am also amazed at how easy it was to stop this unhelpful empty calorie intake by a eating a good filling breakfast.

Objections:

'I am not hungry in the morning'.

Is this true? Or are you so rushed in the morning that you just have got into the habit of not listening to the hunger signals from your tummy? Also, breakfast in the one occasion when you should not rely on the principle *only eat when you are hungry in your stomach (tummy hungry).*

You should eat breakfast every day, irrespective of how you feel. Eventually, starting your day with breakfast will become a good habit.

'I would rather have 10 minutes longer in bed in the morning'.

This is understandable, especially on a cold dark winter morning. However; think about your overall health and wellbeing - Do you really want to achieve and maintain your ideal healthy weight?

You have established your morning routine – a habit. You can change this habit and create a new morning routine that will make you feel better in the long run. The good news is that you do not need to make a radical change. I know because I have done it and I am so glad that I did. In the beginning you only need to sacrifice a few minutes of your precious snooze time.

'I drink coffee and this gives me the boost I need to get started and keep going'.

Coffee certainly does give you a 'kick start'. The problem is this is only a short lived boost – it does not sustain you. You will find yourself needing another boost within a short space of time – and you will probably eat at mid-morning tea-break.

In contrast, the slow release energy achieved by eating a good breakfast, such as porridge, is a much better option in terms of weight management and providing energy, as it will help to maintain your energy levels all morning and keep you feeling fuller-for-longer. This means that you won't need to eat at mid-morning tea-break (as long as you don't eat out of habit).

'I have three children to get ready for school and must get myself ready and out to work,'

Of course it is difficult, but it is not necessarily impossible for you to make the time to fit in breakfast.

You have established a routine which does not include breakfast; however, it may be possible for you to reorganise your routine to include breakfast. It requires a few minutes and you will reap massive benefits. However, if you just cannot get the time to eat before you leave the house, then the next paragraph is for you.

Take it with you, if you can.

Lack of time is not really a good excuse for many of us, because we *can* change our morning routine; however, we live in the real world, and some people may be in circumstances which cannot be adapted easily to fit in breakfast.

If you really cannot make the time to take breakfast before you go to work, why not take it with you in a container and eat it at your workplace before you start your duties?

Alternatively, if you just can't eat breakfast despite your best efforts, perhaps you could take your healthy breakfast at mid-morning tea-break instead of biscuits or chocolate bars. This is not the number one option, as you can't really beat a proper breakfast, but it is better than nothing.

Porridge

If breakfast were an Olympic sport, Porridge would win the gold medal! It is great for filling your tummy in the morning and fuelling you throughout the day.

Warning: Please don't immediately switch off and decide that there is no way that you can take porridge because you don't like the taste or it is too boring. This was my reaction; however, I have made discoveries which have changed my mind.

Excuse busters:

'I don't like porridge'.

I am delighted to say that there is now a wide variety of flavours to choose from and there will be one to suit your particular taste – the day of bland boring porridge is now over!

Also, you can make your morning porridge more interesting by adding various additional items to make it more appealing to your individual taste. For example, you could try adding things such as various types of fruit, honey or nuts, or mix in other healthy breakfast cereals, etc.

'I don't have time in the morning to stand over a saucepan on the cooker and heat a pot of porridge'.

You don't have to cook in a saucepan on the cooker any more, as you can buy porridge that can be cooked in the microwave in *two minutes* – you can even measure the exact amount of milk that you need using the sachet the porridge comes in. I now have a routine established and I make my porridge in the microwave for two minutes at the same time as I put the kettle on for tea.

The science of porridge.

There are many great things in porridge, such as vitamin E, B, folic acid, etc. However, the key ingredient is *oats*.

The oats contain a fibre called *'Beta Glucan'*. This is a *soluble* fibre, which means it dissolves in water and forms a thick mass. This sits in your tummy for longer, thus making you feel fuller-for-longer and switches off the hunger hormone (Ghrelin).

This will help you stop snacking! It also provides the body with fuel at a steadier rate, which will help you work harder for longer and improve concentration.

Every child should fuel up on porridge before they go to school as this could help their academic performance.

Also, the oats undergo minimal processing when the porridge is being produced, thus little natural goodness is lost in the processing process. This is an advantage over other more highly processed breakfast cereals.

Research suggests that Beta Glucan can help lower cholesterol and help protect against heart disease and cancer, as well as helping us manage our weight.

It is interesting to note that porridge is the breakfast of choice for many athletes who take part in a variety of sports, such as: marathon runners and athletes competing in the various track and field events; top cyclists who ride in the events such as the 'Tour de France'; top rowers and professional boxers, etc. Many leading people in the public eye, successful business people and celebrities eat porridge as an essential part of their diet.

Other Breakfast options

Maybe, after your best efforts, you just can't get into the habit of eating porridge, despite the wide range of flavours and very convenient cooking options. Never mind, there are other healthy breakfast options available for you to choose from.

Warning:

Remember to choose your breakfast cereal carefully. Be aware that many are *full of sugar* which is not very helpful if you are managing your weight.

Also, they might not fill your tummy and thus you run the risk of becoming hungry again sooner and become tempted to eat again at mid-morning tea-break.

You are an intelligent person and the key is to use your common sense when you are choosing a breakfast cereal which is consistent with your weight management and healthy lifestyle options.

PART TWO

WHAT YOU NEED TO DO -
TO LOSE WEIGHT AND KEEP IT OFF PERMANENTLY

WITHOUT GOING ON A DIET

Part Two

Contents

Introduction

Time for action

In the previous section we looked at what you need to ***know*** about weight loss.

Now it is time to look in more detail at what you need to ***do*** in order to lose weight, and keep the weight off permanently – *without going on a diet!*

You are going to re-educate yourself to move away from the old bad eating habits that led to you having a weight problem, and establish new natural eating habits.

Remember, this is *not a diet programme*. Rather, it is a *framework* for you to follow.

Chapter 20

The Foundation Stage

You are now entering the foundation stage of your journey into permanent weight loss the natural way '*without going on a diet*'!

Key points:

You do ***not*** change ***what*** you eat during this stage. You will keep eating the foods that you are currently eating.

This is not a diet programme telling you what to cut out, how many calories you should take each day, etc.

At this first stage, you will be changing ***how*** you eat. In other words, you are beginning to learn new natural eating habits to replace the old habits that resulted in your weight gain.

You continue to eat the same food you are consuming at present; however, you will be following the 'Three Point Plan':

1. Eat only when you are genuinely hungry - in your stomach, not your imagination (or 'tummy hungry' to use the old well known phrase).

Learn to 'listen' to your body when it releases the hunger hormone (Ghrelin), to let you know it is time to eat and 're-fuel' your body with food.

2. Eat slowly and enjoy each mouthful.

Slow down, chew your food slowly and do not scoff the food down – as you may have been told as a child.

3. Stop eating when you feel that your stomach feels full.

Learn to 'listen' to your body when it naturally sends the chemical (Leptin) to let you know your stomach it is full.

Key points to remember:

Don't lose too much weight too soon.

You should *not* lose any more than *2 pounds* per week.

Remember, you are gradually re-educating yourself to develop natural eating habits and this will take time. It is important to be patient because true, permanent weight loss takes time.

If you lose too much weight too soon, you will go into *'famine mode'*. This will defeat the purpose of this weight loss programme because you will be 'on a diet' and not permanently re-educating your eating habits.

Don't weigh yourself every day or every week.

It is important that you do not weigh yourself too often. I suggest that you should stand on the scales once every three weeks in the early stages of this programme.

You may find it helpful to use the 'review day and progress check' pages of the 'full support framework' in chapters 22 – 24, at the designated time.

Let your clothes be your guide.

If you follow this approach to weight loss, you will notice that your clothes gradually begin to become loose.

Do not obsessively count calories at this stage.

Remember, this is not a diet plan. You are beginning to change your eating habits.

There are no 'banned' foods at this stage.

This is not a diet plan. At this stage you are not 'cutting out' food items. You are changing **how** you eat (re-educating your eating habits).

Once you start to re-educate your eating habits, you should find that you will naturally stop wanting the unhealthy foods that are such an enemy of your waistline.

I loved chocolate and cream cakes and did not ever think that I would ever be able to resist eating these items. Certainly willpower did not work.

By following the natural weight loss approach outlined in this book, I can enjoy these food items but I am no longer controlled by the same strong desire – I am in control! Do I still eat chocolate and cream cakes? Yes! Am I addicted to chocolate and cream cakes? No! I will eat and enjoy a bar of chocolate or a cream cake *occasionally.*

The key difference is I am now in control because my eating habits have been re-educated.

This is easier than ‘cutting out’ as part of a diet - the results will be real and permanent.

Chapter 21

Foundation stage: ***A summary card***

You may find it helpful to have a simple visual prompt to help keep you on track as you work to re-educate your eating habits.

I have provided a summary card in this chapter for you to photocopy and carry in your pocket or handbag, pin up in your kitchen or, workplace, etc.

This will act as a *'prompt card'* to help you stick to the principles of 'Three Point Plan'.

Maybe you don't need this, but you may find it helpful refer to it when you are going to eat, and are trying to decide if it is true physical hunger in your stomach ('tummy hunger') or hunger in your imagination ('head hunger').

Additionally, you may find it helpful to have a *full programme framework* to follow to help to keep you on track.

This framework consists of *'daily prompt cards'* to help you stick to the principles of the 'Three Point Plan'

If so, I have provided such a framework of 'prompt cards' for you to follow in the subsequent chapters, should you require them.

Summary Card

Follow the 'Three Point Plan'.

1. Eat only when you are genuinely hungry in your *stomach* and not in your imagination (when the hunger hormone *Ghrelin* indicates that your body needs 'fuel').

.

2. Eat slowly.

3. Stop eating when your stomach signals that it is *full* (when *Leptin* is released to indicate that your body has had enough 'fuel').

Breakfast	Did you have a healthy filling breakfast? Yes ( ) No ( )
Mid-morning snack	Are you tummy hungry? Do you need to eat? Yes ( ) No ( )
Lunch	Did you follow the 'Three Point Plan'? Yes ( ) No ( )
Mid-afternoon snack	Are you tummy hungry? Do you need to eat? Yes ( ) No ( )
Evening meal	Did you follow the 'Three Point Plan'? Yes ( ) No ( )
Snack: watching TV movie, etc.,	Are you tummy hungry? Do you need to eat? Yes ( ) No ( )
Bedtime snack / supper	Are you tummy hungry? Do you need to eat? Yes ( ) No ( )

Exercise: Did you do something to make your heart beat faster?
Walking ( ) Other ( )

Chapter 22

Daily programme: Foundation stage *Phase 1*

You may find it helpful to have a full support programme framework to follow in order to help you re-educate your eating habits.

This is ***not a diet plan*** telling you which food items you *should* or *shouldn't* eat.

It is a ***framework,*** with ***'daily prompt cards'*** to help you stick to the principles of *'Three Point Plan'*.

How to use your '*daily prompt cards*':

- Keep the book in a convenient location for quick reference to the prompt cards throughout the day.

- Follow the cards in the correct order and write the date on the appropriate page. This will help you keep track of your progress.

- Read them at the relevant time of the day. For example, at morning tea-break time, read and complete the section: '*Mid-morning snack*'.

- If you feel hungry outside the times listed on the cards, use them to help you decide if you are: *genuinely* hungry in your *stomach* (when the hunger hormone *Ghrelin* indicates that your body needs 'fuel') and not in your *imagination.*

Daily programme: Foundation stage *Phase 1.*

Change eating habits Support Plan & Progress tracker

This part of the plan will last for ***3 weeks***.

You will weigh yourself on **Day 1** (you will *not* use the scales until the end of week 3).

You will weigh yourself again at the ***end of week 3.***

The plan is divided into the following weekly elements:

Day 1 – 5 (Monday – Friday*): Main programme.

Day 6: Treat day.

Day 7: In-between 'balance' day.

*If you work shift patterns which involve weekend work – no problem. Fit the 5 day main programme plan into your weekly schedule.

Please have faith in the plan and keep going and you should see results. It will take time, but it will be worth it as the weight loss will be real, natural and permanent.

Don't forget:

You should make sure that you try to do some 'Level A' exercise every day.

Foundation Phase 1
Week 1

Day 1 **Date** ________

Follow the 'Three Point Plan'.

1. Eat only when you are genuinely hungry in your *stomach* and not in your imagination (when the hunger hormone *Ghrelin* indicates that your body needs 'fuel').

.
2. Eat slowly.

3. Stop eating when your stomach signals that it is *full* (when *Leptin* is released to indicate that your body has had enough 'fuel').

Breakfast	Did you have a healthy filling breakfast? Yes ( ) No ( )
Mid-morning snack	Are you tummy hungry? Do you need to eat? Yes ( ) No ( )
Lunch	Did you follow the 'Three Point Plan'? Yes ( ) No ( )
Mid-afternoon snack	Are you tummy hungry? Do you need to eat? Yes ( ) No ( )
Evening meal	Did you follow the 'Three Point Plan'? Yes ( ) No ( )
Snack: watching TV movie, etc.,	Are you tummy hungry? Do you need to eat? Yes ( ) No ( )
Bedtime snack / supper	Are you tummy hungry? Do you need to eat? Yes ( ) No ( )

Exercise: Did you do something to make your heart beat faster?
Walking ( ) Other ( )

Foundation Phase 1
Week 1

Day 2 **Date** ________

Follow the 'Three Point Plan'.

1. Eat only when you are genuinely hungry in your *stomach* and not in your imagination (when the hunger hormone *Ghrelin* indicates that your body needs 'fuel').

.

2. Eat slowly.

3. Stop eating when your stomach signals that it is *full* (when *Leptin* is released to indicate that your body has had enough 'fuel').

Breakfast	Did you have a healthy filling breakfast? Yes ( ) No ( )
Mid-morning snack	Are you tummy hungry? Do you need to eat? Yes ( ) No ( )
Lunch	Did you follow the 'Three Point Plan'? Yes ( ) No ( )
Mid-afternoon snack	Are you tummy hungry? Do you need to eat? Yes ( ) No ( )
Evening meal	Did you follow the 'Three Point Plan'? Yes ( ) No ( )
Snack: watching TV movie, etc.,	Are you tummy hungry? Do you need to eat? Yes ( ) No ( )
Bedtime snack / supper	Are you tummy hungry? Do you need to eat? Yes ( ) No ( )

Exercise: Did you do something to make your heart beat faster?
Walking ( ) Other ( )

Foundation Phase 1
Week 1

Day 3 **Date ________**

Follow the 'Three Point Plan'.

1. Eat only when you are genuinely hungry in your *stomach* and not in your imagination (when the hunger hormone *Ghrelin* indicates that your body needs 'fuel').

.

2. Eat slowly.

3. Stop eating when your stomach signals that it is *full* (when *Leptin* is released to indicate that your body has had enough 'fuel').

Breakfast	Did you have a healthy filling breakfast? Yes ( ) No ( )
Mid-morning snack	Are you tummy hungry? Do you need to eat? Yes ( ) No ( )
Lunch	Did you follow the 'Three Point Plan'? Yes ( ) No ( )
Mid-afternoon snack	Are you tummy hungry? Do you need to eat? Yes ( ) No ( )
Evening meal	Did you follow the 'Three Point Plan'? Yes ( ) No ( )
Snack: watching TV movie, etc.,	Are you tummy hungry? Do you need to eat? Yes ( ) No ( )
Bedtime snack / supper	Are you tummy hungry? Do you need to eat? Yes ( ) No ( )

Exercise: Did you do something to make your heart beat faster?
Walking ( ) Other ( )

Foundation Phase 1
Week 1

Day 4 **Date ________**

<table>
<tr><td colspan="2">Follow the 'Three Point Plan'.

1. Eat only when you are genuinely hungry in your stomach and not in your imagination (when the hunger hormone Ghrelin indicates that your body needs 'fuel').
.
2. Eat slowly.

3. Stop eating when your stomach signals that it is full (when Leptin is released to indicate that your body has had enough 'fuel').</td></tr>
<tr><td>Breakfast</td><td>Did you have a healthy filling breakfast?
Yes ( ) No ( )</td></tr>
<tr><td>Mid-morning snack</td><td>Are you tummy hungry?
Do you need to eat?
Yes ( ) No ( )</td></tr>
<tr><td>Lunch</td><td>Did you follow the 'Three Point Plan'?
Yes ( ) No ( )</td></tr>
<tr><td>Mid-afternoon snack</td><td>Are you tummy hungry?
Do you need to eat?
Yes ( ) No ( )</td></tr>
<tr><td>Evening meal</td><td>Did you follow the 'Three Point Plan'?
Yes ( ) No ( )</td></tr>
<tr><td>Snack: watching TV movie, etc.,</td><td>Are you tummy hungry?
Do you need to eat?
Yes ( ) No ( )</td></tr>
<tr><td>Bedtime snack / supper</td><td>Are you tummy hungry?
Do you need to eat?
Yes ( ) No ( )</td></tr>
</table>

Exercise: Did you do something to make your heart beat faster?
Walking ( ) Other ( )

Foundation Phase 1
Week 1

Day 5 **Date ________**

Follow the 'Three Point Plan'. **1. Eat only when you are genuinely hungry in your *stomach* and not in your imagination** (when the hunger hormone *Ghrelin* indicates that your body needs 'fuel'). . **2. Eat slowly.** **3. Stop eating when your stomach signals that it is *full*** (when *Leptin* is released to indicate that your body has had enough 'fuel').	
Breakfast	Did you have a healthy filling breakfast? Yes ( ) No ( )
Mid-morning snack	Are you tummy hungry? Do you need to eat? Yes ( ) No ( )
Lunch	Did you follow the 'Three Point Plan'? Yes ( ) No ( )
Mid-afternoon snack	Are you tummy hungry? Do you need to eat? Yes ( ) No ( )
Evening meal	Did you follow the 'Three Point Plan'? Yes ( ) No ( )
Snack: watching TV movie, etc.,	Are you tummy hungry? Do you need to eat? Yes ( ) No ( )
Bedtime snack / supper	Are you tummy hungry? Do you need to eat? Yes ( ) No ( )

Exercise: Did you do something to make your heart beat faster?
Walking ( ) Other ( )

Foundation Phase 1
Week 1

Day 6 **Date ________**

'Treat Day'.

Eat whatever you want and enjoy.

As you continue to follow this plan, you will find that you will gradually change the amount of 'treat' foods you eat.

Day 7 **Date ________**

In-between 'balance' day.

You will try to balance between following the 'Three Point Plan' and eating whatever you want and enjoy.

As you continue to follow this plan, you will find that you will gradually change the amount of 'treat' foods you eat.

Please keep faith in the plan.

Keep going and you will see real results.

Foundation Phase 1
Week 2

Day 1 **Date ________**

Follow the 'Three Point Plan'.

1. Eat only when you are genuinely hungry in your *stomach* and not in your imagination (when the hunger hormone *Ghrelin* indicates that your body needs 'fuel').

.

2. Eat slowly.

3. Stop eating when your stomach signals that it is *full* (when *Leptin* is released to indicate that your body has had enough 'fuel').

Breakfast	Did you have a healthy filling breakfast? Yes ( ) No ( )
Mid-morning snack	Are you tummy hungry? Do you need to eat? Yes ( ) No ( )
Lunch	Did you follow the 'Three Point Plan'? Yes ( ) No ( )
Mid-afternoon snack	Are you tummy hungry? Do you need to eat? Yes ( ) No ( )
Evening meal	Did you follow the 'Three Point Plan'? Yes ( ) No ( )
Snack: watching TV movie, etc.,	Are you tummy hungry? Do you need to eat? Yes ( ) No ( )
Bedtime snack / supper	Are you tummy hungry? Do you need to eat? Yes ( ) No ( )

Exercise: Did you do something to make your heart beat faster?
Walking ( ) Other ( )

Foundation Phase 1
Week 2

Day 2 **Date ________**

<table>
<tr><td colspan="2">Follow the 'Three Point Plan'.

1. Eat only when you are genuinely hungry in your stomach and not in your imagination (when the hunger hormone Ghrelin indicates that your body needs 'fuel').
.
2. Eat slowly.

3. Stop eating when your stomach signals that it is full (when Leptin is released to indicate that your body has had enough 'fuel').</td></tr>
<tr><td>Breakfast</td><td>Did you have a healthy filling breakfast?
Yes ( ) No ( )</td></tr>
<tr><td>Mid-morning snack</td><td>Are you tummy hungry?
Do you need to eat?
Yes ( ) No ( )</td></tr>
<tr><td>Lunch</td><td>Did you follow the 'Three Point Plan'?
Yes ( ) No ( )</td></tr>
<tr><td>Mid-afternoon snack</td><td>Are you tummy hungry?
Do you need to eat?
Yes ( ) No ( )</td></tr>
<tr><td>Evening meal</td><td>Did you follow the 'Three Point Plan'?
Yes ( ) No ( )</td></tr>
<tr><td>Snack: watching TV movie, etc.,</td><td>Are you tummy hungry?
Do you need to eat?
Yes ( ) No ( )</td></tr>
<tr><td>Bedtime snack / supper</td><td>Are you tummy hungry?
Do you need to eat?
Yes ( ) No ( )</td></tr>
</table>

Exercise: Did you do something to make your heart beat faster?
Walking ( ) Other ( )

Foundation Phase 1
Week 2

Day 3 **Date ________**

<table>
<tr><td colspan="2">Follow the 'Three Point Plan'.

1. Eat only when you are genuinely hungry in your stomach and not in your imagination (when the hunger hormone Ghrelin indicates that your body needs 'fuel').
.
2. Eat slowly.

3. Stop eating when your stomach signals that it is full (when Leptin is released to indicate that your body has had enough 'fuel').</td></tr>
<tr><td>Breakfast</td><td>Did you have a healthy filling breakfast?
Yes ( ) No ( )</td></tr>
<tr><td>Mid-morning snack</td><td>Are you tummy hungry?
Do you need to eat?
Yes ( ) No ( )</td></tr>
<tr><td>Lunch</td><td>Did you follow the 'Three Point Plan'?
Yes ( ) No ( )</td></tr>
<tr><td>Mid-afternoon snack</td><td>Are you tummy hungry?
Do you need to eat?
Yes ( ) No ( )</td></tr>
<tr><td>Evening meal</td><td>Did you follow the 'Three Point Plan'?
Yes ( ) No ( )</td></tr>
<tr><td>Snack: watching TV movie, etc.,</td><td>Are you tummy hungry?
Do you need to eat?
Yes ( ) No ( )</td></tr>
<tr><td>Bedtime snack / supper</td><td>Are you tummy hungry?
Do you need to eat?
Yes ( ) No ( )</td></tr>
</table>

Exercise: Did you do something to make your heart beat faster?
Walking ( ) Other ( )

Foundation Phase 1
Week 2

Day 4 **Date ________**

<table>
<tr><td colspan="2">Follow the 'Three Point Plan'.

1. Eat only when you are genuinely hungry in your stomach and not in your imagination (when the hunger hormone Ghrelin indicates that your body needs 'fuel').
.
2. Eat slowly.

3. Stop eating when your stomach signals that it is full (when Leptin is released to indicate that your body has had enough 'fuel').</td></tr>
<tr><td>Breakfast</td><td>Did you have a healthy filling breakfast?
Yes ( ) No ( )</td></tr>
<tr><td>Mid-morning snack</td><td>Are you tummy hungry?
Do you need to eat?
Yes ( ) No ( )</td></tr>
<tr><td>Lunch</td><td>Did you follow the 'Three Point Plan'?
Yes ( ) No ( )</td></tr>
<tr><td>Mid-afternoon snack</td><td>Are you tummy hungry?
Do you need to eat?
Yes ( ) No ( )</td></tr>
<tr><td>Evening meal</td><td>Did you follow the 'Three Point Plan'?
Yes ( ) No ( )</td></tr>
<tr><td>Snack: watching TV movie, etc.,</td><td>Are you tummy hungry?
Do you need to eat?
Yes ( ) No ( )</td></tr>
<tr><td>Bedtime snack / supper</td><td>Are you tummy hungry?
Do you need to eat?
Yes ( ) No ( )</td></tr>
</table>

Exercise: Did you do something to make your heart beat faster?
Walking ( ) Other ( )

Foundation Phase 1
Week 2

Day 5 **Date** ________

<table>
<tr><td colspan="2">Follow the 'Three Point Plan'.

1. Eat only when you are genuinely hungry in your stomach and not in your imagination (when the hunger hormone Ghrelin indicates that your body needs 'fuel').
.
2. Eat slowly.

3. Stop eating when your stomach signals that it is full (when Leptin is released to indicate that your body has had enough 'fuel').</td></tr>
<tr><td>Breakfast</td><td>Did you have a healthy filling breakfast?
Yes ( ) No ( )</td></tr>
<tr><td>Mid-morning snack</td><td>Are you tummy hungry?
Do you need to eat?
Yes ( ) No ( )</td></tr>
<tr><td>Lunch</td><td>Did you follow the 'Three Point Plan'?
Yes ( ) No ( )</td></tr>
<tr><td>Mid-afternoon snack</td><td>Are you tummy hungry?
Do you need to eat?
Yes ( ) No ( )</td></tr>
<tr><td>Evening meal</td><td>Did you follow the 'Three Point Plan'?
Yes ( ) No ( )</td></tr>
<tr><td>Snack: watching TV movie, etc.,</td><td>Are you tummy hungry?
Do you need to eat?
Yes ( ) No ( )</td></tr>
<tr><td>Bedtime snack / supper</td><td>Are you tummy hungry?
Do you need to eat?
Yes ( ) No ( )</td></tr>
</table>

Exercise: Did you do something to make your heart beat faster?
Walking ( ) Other ( )

Foundation Phase 1
Week 2

Day 6 **Date ________**

'Treat Day'

Eat whatever you want and enjoy.

As you continue to follow this plan, you will find that you will gradually change the amount of 'treat' foods you eat.

Day 7 **Date ________**

In-between 'balance' day.

You will try to balance between following the 'Three Point Plan' and eating whatever you want and enjoy.

As you continue to follow this plan, you will find that you will gradually change the amount of 'treat' foods you eat.

Please keep faith in the plan.

Keep going and you will see real results.

Foundation Phase 1
Week 3

Day 1 **Date** ________

<table>
<tr><td colspan="2">Follow the 'Three Point Plan'.

1. Eat only when you are genuinely hungry in your *stomach* and not in your imagination (when the hunger hormone *Ghrelin* indicates that your body needs 'fuel').
.
2. Eat slowly.

3. Stop eating when your stomach signals that it is *full* (when *Leptin* is released to indicate that your body has had enough 'fuel').</td></tr>
<tr><td>Breakfast</td><td>Did you have a healthy filling breakfast?
Yes ( ) No ( )</td></tr>
<tr><td>Mid-morning snack</td><td>Are you tummy hungry?
Do you need to eat?
Yes ( ) No ( )</td></tr>
<tr><td>Lunch</td><td>Did you follow the 'Three Point Plan'?
Yes ( ) No ( )</td></tr>
<tr><td>Mid-afternoon snack</td><td>Are you tummy hungry?
Do you need to eat?
Yes ( ) No ( )</td></tr>
<tr><td>Evening meal</td><td>Did you follow the 'Three Point Plan'?
Yes ( ) No ( )</td></tr>
<tr><td>Snack: watching TV movie, etc.,</td><td>Are you tummy hungry?
Do you need to eat?
Yes ( ) No ( )</td></tr>
<tr><td>Bedtime snack / supper</td><td>Are you tummy hungry?
Do you need to eat?
Yes ( ) No ( )</td></tr>
</table>

Exercise: Did you do something to make your heart beat faster?
Walking ( ) Other ( )

Foundation Phase 1
Week 3

Day 2 **Date** ________

Follow the 'Three Point Plan'. **1. Eat only when you are genuinely hungry in your *stomach* and not in your imagination** (when the hunger hormone *Ghrelin* indicates that your body needs 'fuel'). . **2. Eat slowly.** **3. Stop eating when your stomach signals that it is *full*** (when *Leptin* is released to indicate that your body has had enough 'fuel').	
Breakfast	Did you have a healthy filling breakfast? Yes ( ) No ( )
Mid-morning snack	Are you tummy hungry? Do you need to eat? Yes ( ) No ( )
Lunch	Did you follow the 'Three Point Plan'? Yes ( ) No ( )
Mid-afternoon snack	Are you tummy hungry? Do you need to eat? Yes ( ) No ( )
Evening meal	Did you follow the 'Three Point Plan'? Yes ( ) No ( )
Snack: watching TV movie, etc.,	Are you tummy hungry? Do you need to eat? Yes ( ) No ( )
Bedtime snack / supper	Are you tummy hungry? Do you need to eat? Yes ( ) No ( )

Exercise: Did you do something to make your heart beat faster?
Walking ( ) Other ( )

Foundation Phase 1
Week 3

Day 3 **Date ________**

<table>
<tr><td colspan="2">Follow the 'Three Point Plan'.

1. Eat only when you are genuinely hungry in your stomach and not in your imagination (when the hunger hormone Ghrelin indicates that your body needs 'fuel').
.
2. Eat slowly.

3. Stop eating when your stomach signals that it is full (when Leptin is released to indicate that your body has had enough 'fuel').</td></tr>
<tr><td>Breakfast</td><td>Did you have a healthy filling breakfast?
Yes ( ) No ( )</td></tr>
<tr><td>Mid-morning snack</td><td>Are you tummy hungry?
Do you need to eat?
Yes ( ) No ( )</td></tr>
<tr><td>Lunch</td><td>Did you follow the 'Three Point Plan'?
Yes ( ) No ( )</td></tr>
<tr><td>Mid-afternoon snack</td><td>Are you tummy hungry?
Do you need to eat?
Yes ( ) No ( )</td></tr>
<tr><td>Evening meal</td><td>Did you follow the 'Three Point Plan'?
Yes ( ) No ( )</td></tr>
<tr><td>Snack: watching TV movie, etc.,</td><td>Are you tummy hungry?
Do you need to eat?
Yes ( ) No ( )</td></tr>
<tr><td>Bedtime snack / supper</td><td>Are you tummy hungry?
Do you need to eat?
Yes ( ) No ( )</td></tr>
</table>

Exercise: Did you do something to make your heart beat faster?
Walking ( ) Other ( )

Foundation Phase 1

Week 3

Day 4 **Date ________**

<table>
<tr><td colspan="2">Follow the 'Three Point Plan'.

1. Eat only when you are genuinely hungry in your *stomach* and not in your imagination (when the hunger hormone *Ghrelin* indicates that your body needs 'fuel').
.
2. Eat slowly.

3. Stop eating when your stomach signals that it is *full* (when *Leptin* is released to indicate that your body has had enough 'fuel').</td></tr>
<tr><td>Breakfast</td><td>Did you have a healthy filling breakfast?
Yes ( ) No ( )</td></tr>
<tr><td>Mid-morning snack</td><td>Are you tummy hungry?
Do you need to eat?
Yes ( ) No ( )</td></tr>
<tr><td>Lunch</td><td>Did you follow the 'Three Point Plan'?
Yes ( ) No ( )</td></tr>
<tr><td>Mid-afternoon snack</td><td>Are you tummy hungry?
Do you need to eat?
Yes ( ) No ( )</td></tr>
<tr><td>Evening meal</td><td>Did you follow the 'Three Point Plan'?
Yes ( ) No ( )</td></tr>
<tr><td>Snack: watching TV movie, etc.,</td><td>Are you tummy hungry?
Do you need to eat?
Yes ( ) No ( )</td></tr>
<tr><td>Bedtime snack / supper</td><td>Are you tummy hungry?
Do you need to eat?
Yes ( ) No ( )</td></tr>
</table>

Exercise: Did you do something to make your heart beat faster?
Walking ( ) Other ( )

Foundation Phase 1
Week 3

Day 5 **Date ________**

Follow the 'Three Point Plan'.

1. Eat only when you are genuinely hungry in your *stomach* and not in your imagination (when the hunger hormone *Ghrelin* indicates that your body needs 'fuel').

.

2. Eat slowly.

3. Stop eating when your stomach signals that it is *full* (when *Leptin* is released to indicate that your body has had enough 'fuel').

Breakfast	Did you have a healthy filling breakfast? Yes ( ) No ( )
Mid-morning snack	Are you tummy hungry? Do you need to eat? Yes ( ) No ( )
Lunch	Did you follow the 'Three Point Plan'? Yes ( ) No ( )
Mid-afternoon snack	Are you tummy hungry? Do you need to eat? Yes ( ) No ( )
Evening meal	Did you follow the 'Three Point Plan'? Yes ( ) No ( )
Snack: watching TV movie, etc.,	Are you tummy hungry? Do you need to eat? Yes ( ) No ( )
Bedtime snack / supper	Are you tummy hungry? Do you need to eat? Yes ( ) No ( )

Exercise: Did you do something to make your heart beat faster?
Walking ( ) Other ( )

Foundation Phase 1
Week 3

Day 6 **Date ________**

'Treat Day'

Eat whatever you want and enjoy.

As you continue to follow this plan, you will find that you will gradually change the amount of 'treat' foods you eat.

Day 7 **Date ________**

In-between 'balance' day.

You will try to balance between following the 'Three Point Plan' and eating whatever you want and enjoy.

As you continue to follow this plan, you will find that you will gradually change the amount of 'treat' foods you eat.

Please keep faith in the plan.

Keep going and you will see real results.

Please complete the 'Review and progress check' on the next page.

Foundation Phase 1
Week 3

Day 7 **Date ________**

Review day and progress check.

Today is the day that you will stand on the scales and review your progress.

To achieve the most accurate weight, I suggest that you follow the procedure stated below.

- Weigh yourself first thing in the morning before breakfast.
- Wear as few clothes as possible (if any).
- Make sure the scales are set at zero.
- Stand on the correct part of the scale – see the manufacturer's instructions if you are not sure.
- Take three readings – they should all be the same. If you do get different readings, make sure that the scale is reset to zero before each reading.
- Write down the answer.
- Be honest and write down the true weight reading, not what you want the scales to say.

You may find it helpful to record the result below.

Weight: ____________

Weight lost: ___________

Did you lose any weight? Yes ( ) No ( )

If **yes**: well done and keep up the good work. You are re-educating your eating habits and are well on the way to achieving your weight loss goals.

Remember, you should aim to lose between 1 – 2 pounds per week.

If **no**: don't be discouraged. Ask yourself why - did you really follow the 'Three Point Plan' required for natural weight loss?

I know from my personal experience of following this plan that you can lose weight if you stick to the requirements of the programme. Start to follow the programme again and you should lose weight – if you follow the plan!

Well done!

You have completed *Phase 1* of the foundation stage of your weight loss journey.

It is now time to build upon your success in the first phase. You shall now continue to establish the eating habits required to help you achieve and maintain your ideal natural weight.

Chapter 23

Daily programme: Foundation stage *Phase 2*

Change eating habits Support Plan & Progress tracker

This part of the plan will last for ***3 weeks***.

You will weigh yourself on **Day 1** (you will *not* use the scales until the end of week 3).

You will weigh yourself again at the ***end of week 3.***

The plan is divided into the following weekly elements:

Day 1 – 5 (Monday – Friday*): Main programme.

Day 6: Treat day.

Day 7: In-between 'balance' day.

*If you work shift patterns which involve weekend work – no problem. Fit the 5 day main programme plan into your weekly schedule.

Please have faith in the plan and keep going and you should see results. It will take time, but it will be worth it as the weight loss will be real, natural and permanent.

Don't forget: You should make sure that you try to do some 'Level A' exercise every day.

Foundation Phase 2
Week 1

Day 1 **Date ________**

Follow the 'Three Point Plan'. **1. Eat only when you are genuinely hungry in your *stomach* and not in your imagination** (when the hunger hormone *Ghrelin* indicates that your body needs 'fuel'). . **2. Eat slowly.** **3. Stop eating when your stomach signals that it is *full*** (when *Leptin* is released to indicate that your body has had enough 'fuel').	
Breakfast	Did you have a healthy filling breakfast? Yes ( ) No ( )
Mid-morning snack	Are you tummy hungry? Do you need to eat? Yes ( ) No ( )
Lunch	Did you follow the 'Three Point Plan'? Yes ( ) No ( )
Mid-afternoon snack	Are you tummy hungry? Do you need to eat? Yes ( ) No ( )
Evening meal	Did you follow the 'Three Point Plan'? Yes ( ) No ( )
Snack: watching TV movie, etc.,	Are you tummy hungry? Do you need to eat? Yes ( ) No ( )
Bedtime snack / supper	Are you tummy hungry? Do you need to eat? Yes ( ) No ( )

Exercise: Did you do something to make your heart beat faster?
Walking ( ) Other ( )

Foundation Phase 2
Week 1

Day 2 **Date** ________

Follow the 'Three Point Plan'. **1. Eat only when you are genuinely hungry in your *stomach* and not in your imagination** (when the hunger hormone *Ghrelin* indicates that your body needs 'fuel'). . **2. Eat slowly.** **3. Stop eating when your stomach signals that it is *full*** (when *Leptin* is released to indicate that your body has had enough 'fuel').	
Breakfast	Did you have a healthy filling breakfast? Yes ( ) No ( )
Mid-morning snack	Are you tummy hungry? Do you need to eat? Yes ( ) No ( )
Lunch	Did you follow the 'Three Point Plan'? Yes ( ) No ( )
Mid-afternoon snack	Are you tummy hungry? Do you need to eat? Yes ( ) No ( )
Evening meal	Did you follow the 'Three Point Plan'? Yes ( ) No ( )
Snack: watching TV movie, etc.,	Are you tummy hungry? Do you need to eat? Yes ( ) No ( )
Bedtime snack / supper	Are you tummy hungry? Do you need to eat? Yes ( ) No ( )

Exercise: Did you do something to make your heart beat faster?
Walking ( ) Other ( )

Foundation Phase 2
Week 1

Day 3 **Date** ________

Follow the 'Three Point Plan'. **1. Eat only when you are genuinely hungry in your *stomach* and not in your imagination** (when the hunger hormone *Ghrelin* indicates that your body needs 'fuel'). . **2. Eat slowly.** **3. Stop eating when your stomach signals that it is *full*** (when *Leptin* is released to indicate that your body has had enough 'fuel').	
Breakfast	Did you have a healthy filling breakfast? Yes ( ) No ( )
Mid-morning snack	Are you tummy hungry? Do you need to eat? Yes ( ) No ( )
Lunch	Did you follow the 'Three Point Plan'? Yes ( ) No ( )
Mid-afternoon snack	Are you tummy hungry? Do you need to eat? Yes ( ) No ( )
Evening meal	Did you follow the 'Three Point Plan'? Yes ( ) No ( )
Snack: watching TV movie, etc.,	Are you tummy hungry? Do you need to eat? Yes ( ) No ( )
Bedtime snack / supper	Are you tummy hungry? Do you need to eat? Yes ( ) No ( )

Exercise: Did you do something to make your heart beat faster?
Walking ( ) Other ( )

Foundation Phase 2
Week 1

Day 4 **Date ________**

Follow the 'Three Point Plan'. **1. Eat only when you are genuinely hungry in your *stomach* and not in your imagination** (when the hunger hormone *Ghrelin* indicates that your body needs 'fuel'). . **2. Eat slowly.** **3. Stop eating when your stomach signals that it is *full*** (when *Leptin* is released to indicate that your body has had enough 'fuel').	
Breakfast	Did you have a healthy filling breakfast? Yes ( ) No ( )
Mid-morning snack	Are you tummy hungry? Do you need to eat? Yes ( ) No ( )
Lunch	Did you follow the 'Three Point Plan'? Yes ( ) No ( )
Mid-afternoon snack	Are you tummy hungry? Do you need to eat? Yes ( ) No ( )
Evening meal	Did you follow the 'Three Point Plan'? Yes ( ) No ( )
Snack: watching TV movie, etc.,	Are you tummy hungry? Do you need to eat? Yes ( ) No ( )
Bedtime snack / supper	Are you tummy hungry? Do you need to eat? Yes ( ) No ( )

Exercise: Did you do something to make your heart beat faster?
Walking ( ) Other ( )

Foundation Phase 2
Week 1

Day 5 **Date ________**

<table>
<tr><td colspan="2">Follow the 'Three Point Plan'.

1. Eat only when you are genuinely hungry in your *stomach* and not in your imagination (when the hunger hormone *Ghrelin* indicates that your body needs 'fuel').
.
2. Eat slowly.

3. Stop eating when your stomach signals that it is *full* (when *Leptin* is released to indicate that your body has had enough 'fuel').</td></tr>
<tr><td>Breakfast</td><td>Did you have a healthy filling breakfast?
Yes ( ) No ( )</td></tr>
<tr><td>Mid-morning snack</td><td>Are you tummy hungry?
Do you need to eat?
Yes ( ) No ( )</td></tr>
<tr><td>Lunch</td><td>Did you follow the 'Three Point Plan'?
Yes ( ) No ( )</td></tr>
<tr><td>Mid-afternoon snack</td><td>Are you tummy hungry?
Do you need to eat?
Yes ( ) No ( )</td></tr>
<tr><td>Evening meal</td><td>Did you follow the 'Three Point Plan'?
Yes ( ) No ( )</td></tr>
<tr><td>Snack: watching TV movie, etc.,</td><td>Are you tummy hungry?
Do you need to eat?
Yes ( ) No ( )</td></tr>
<tr><td>Bedtime snack / supper</td><td>Are you tummy hungry?
Do you need to eat?
Yes ( ) No ( )</td></tr>
</table>

Exercise: Did you do something to make your heart beat faster?
Walking ( ) Other ( )

Foundation Phase 2
Week 1

Day 6 **Date ________**

'Treat Day'

Eat whatever you want and enjoy.

As you continue to follow this plan, you will find that you will gradually change the amount of 'treat' foods you eat.

Day 7 **Date ________**

In-between 'balance' day.

You will try to balance between following the 'Three Point Plan' and eating whatever you want and enjoy.

As you continue to follow this plan, you will find that you will gradually change the amount of 'treat' foods you eat.

Please keep faith in the plan.

Keep going and you will see real results.

Foundation Phase 2
Week 2

Day 1 **Date** ________

Follow the 'Three Point Plan'.

1. Eat only when you are genuinely hungry in your *stomach* and not in your imagination (when the hunger hormone *Ghrelin* indicates that your body needs 'fuel').

.

2. Eat slowly.

3. Stop eating when your stomach signals that it is *full* (when *Leptin* is released to indicate that your body has had enough 'fuel').

Breakfast	Did you have a healthy filling breakfast? Yes ( ) No ( )
Mid-morning snack	Are you tummy hungry? Do you need to eat? Yes ( ) No ( )
Lunch	Did you follow the 'Three Point Plan'? Yes ( ) No ( )
Mid-afternoon snack	Are you tummy hungry? Do you need to eat? Yes ( ) No ( )
Evening meal	Did you follow the 'Three Point Plan'? Yes ( ) No ( )
Snack: watching TV movie, etc.,	Are you tummy hungry? Do you need to eat? Yes ( ) No ( )
Bedtime snack / supper	Are you tummy hungry? Do you need to eat? Yes ( ) No ( )

Exercise: Did you do something to make your heart beat faster?
Walking ( ) Other ( )

Foundation Phase 2
Week 2

Day 2 **Date** ________

Follow the 'Three Point Plan'. **1. Eat only when you are genuinely hungry in your *stomach* and not in your imagination** (when the hunger hormone *Ghrelin* indicates that your body needs 'fuel'). **2. Eat slowly.** **3. Stop eating when your stomach signals that it is *full*** (when *Leptin* is released to indicate that your body has had enough 'fuel').	
Breakfast	Did you have a healthy filling breakfast? Yes ( ) No ( )
Mid-morning snack	Are you tummy hungry? Do you need to eat? Yes ( ) No ( )
Lunch	Did you follow the 'Three Point Plan'? Yes ( ) No ( )
Mid-afternoon snack	Are you tummy hungry? Do you need to eat? Yes ( ) No ( )
Evening meal	Did you follow the 'Three Point Plan'? Yes ( ) No ( )
Snack: watching TV movie, etc.,	Are you tummy hungry? Do you need to eat? Yes ( ) No ( )
Bedtime snack / supper	Are you tummy hungry? Do you need to eat? Yes ( ) No ( )

Exercise: Did you do something to make your heart beat faster?
Walking ( ) Other ( )

Foundation Phase 2
Week 2

Day 3 **Date ________**

Follow the 'Three Point Plan'. **1. Eat only when you are genuinely hungry in your *stomach* and not in your imagination** (when the hunger hormone *Ghrelin* indicates that your body needs 'fuel'). . **2. Eat slowly.** **3. Stop eating when your stomach signals that it is *full*** (when *Leptin* is released to indicate that your body has had enough 'fuel').	
Breakfast	Did you have a healthy filling breakfast? Yes ( ) No ( )
Mid-morning snack	Are you tummy hungry? Do you need to eat? Yes ( ) No ( )
Lunch	Did you follow the 'Three Point Plan'? Yes ( ) No ( )
Mid-afternoon snack	Are you tummy hungry? Do you need to eat? Yes ( ) No ( )
Evening meal	Did you follow the 'Three Point Plan'? Yes ( ) No ( )
Snack: watching TV movie, etc.,	Are you tummy hungry? Do you need to eat? Yes ( ) No ( )
Bedtime snack / supper	Are you tummy hungry? Do you need to eat? Yes ( ) No ( )

Exercise: Did you do something to make your heart beat faster?
Walking ( ) Other ( )

Foundation Phase 2
Week 2

Day 4 **Date ________**

Follow the 'Three Point Plan'.

1. Eat only when you are genuinely hungry in your *stomach* and not in your imagination (when the hunger hormone *Ghrelin* indicates that your body needs 'fuel').

.

2. Eat slowly.

3. Stop eating when your stomach signals that it is *full* (when *Leptin* is released to indicate that your body has had enough 'fuel').

Breakfast	Did you have a healthy filling breakfast? Yes ( ) No ( )
Mid-morning snack	Are you tummy hungry? Do you need to eat? Yes ( ) No ( )
Lunch	Did you follow the 'Three Point Plan'? Yes ( ) No ( )
Mid-afternoon snack	Are you tummy hungry? Do you need to eat? Yes ( ) No ( )
Evening meal	Did you follow the 'Three Point Plan'? Yes ( ) No ( )
Snack: watching TV movie, etc.,	Are you tummy hungry? Do you need to eat? Yes ( ) No ( )
Bedtime snack / supper	Are you tummy hungry? Do you need to eat? Yes ( ) No ( )

Exercise: Did you do something to make your heart beat faster?
Walking ( ) Other ( )

Foundation Phase 2
Week 2

Day 5 **Date ________**

Follow the 'Three Point Plan'.

1. Eat only when you are genuinely hungry in your *stomach* and not in your imagination (when the hunger hormone *Ghrelin* indicates that your body needs 'fuel').

.

2. Eat slowly.

3. Stop eating when your stomach signals that it is *full* (when *Leptin* is released to indicate that your body has had enough 'fuel').

Breakfast	Did you have a healthy filling breakfast? Yes ( ) No ( )
Mid-morning snack	Are you tummy hungry? Do you need to eat? Yes ( ) No ( )
Lunch	Did you follow the 'Three Point Plan'? Yes ( ) No ( )
Mid-afternoon snack	Are you tummy hungry? Do you need to eat? Yes ( ) No ( )
Evening meal	Did you follow the 'Three Point Plan'? Yes ( ) No ( )
Snack: watching TV movie, etc.,	Are you tummy hungry? Do you need to eat? Yes ( ) No ( )
Bedtime snack / supper	Are you tummy hungry? Do you need to eat? Yes ( ) No ( )

Exercise: Did you do something to make your heart beat faster?
Walking ( ) Other ( )

Foundation Phase 2
Week 2

Day 6 **Date ________**

'Treat Day'

Eat whatever you want and enjoy.

As you continue to follow this plan, you will find that you will gradually change the amount of 'treat' foods you eat.

Day 7 **Date ________**

In-between 'balance' day.

You will try to balance between following the 'Three Point Plan' and eating whatever you want and enjoy.

As you continue to follow this plan, you will find that you will gradually change the amount of 'treat' foods you eat.

Please keep faith in the plan.

Keep going and you will see real results.

Foundation Phase 2
Week 3

Day 1 **Date** ________

<table>
<tr><td colspan="2">Follow the 'Three Point Plan'.

1. Eat only when you are genuinely hungry in your *stomach* and not in your imagination (when the hunger hormone *Ghrelin* indicates that your body needs 'fuel').
.
2. Eat slowly.

3. Stop eating when your stomach signals that it is *full* (when *Leptin* is released to indicate that your body has had enough 'fuel').</td></tr>
<tr><td>Breakfast</td><td>Did you have a healthy filling breakfast?
Yes ( ) No ( )</td></tr>
<tr><td>Mid-morning snack</td><td>Are you tummy hungry?
Do you need to eat?
Yes ( ) No ( )</td></tr>
<tr><td>Lunch</td><td>Did you follow the 'Three Point Plan'?
Yes ( ) No ( )</td></tr>
<tr><td>Mid-afternoon snack</td><td>Are you tummy hungry?
Do you need to eat?
Yes ( ) No ( )</td></tr>
<tr><td>Evening meal</td><td>Did you follow the 'Three Point Plan'?
Yes ( ) No ( )</td></tr>
<tr><td>Snack: watching TV movie, etc.,</td><td>Are you tummy hungry?
Do you need to eat?
Yes ( ) No ( )</td></tr>
<tr><td>Bedtime snack / supper</td><td>Are you tummy hungry?
Do you need to eat?
Yes ( ) No ( )</td></tr>
</table>

Exercise: Did you do something to make your heart beat faster?
Walking ( ) Other ( )

Foundation Phase 2
Week 3

Day 2 **Date ________**

Follow the 'Three Point Plan'.

1. Eat only when you are genuinely hungry in your *stomach* and not in your imagination (when the hunger hormone *Ghrelin* indicates that your body needs 'fuel').

.

2. Eat slowly.

3. Stop eating when your stomach signals that it is *full* (when *Leptin* is released to indicate that your body has had enough 'fuel').

Breakfast	Did you have a healthy filling breakfast? Yes ( ) No ( )
Mid-morning snack	Are you tummy hungry? Do you need to eat? Yes ( ) No ( )
Lunch	Did you follow the 'Three Point Plan'? Yes ( ) No ( )
Mid-afternoon snack	Are you tummy hungry? Do you need to eat? Yes ( ) No ( )
Evening meal	Did you follow the 'Three Point Plan'? Yes ( ) No ( )
Snack: watching TV movie, etc.,	Are you tummy hungry? Do you need to eat? Yes ( ) No ( )
Bedtime snack / supper	Are you tummy hungry? Do you need to eat? Yes ( ) No ( )

Exercise: Did you do something to make your heart beat faster?
Walking ( ) Other ( )

Foundation Phase 2
Week 3

Day 3 **Date ________**

<table>
<tr><td colspan="2">Follow the 'Three Point Plan'.

1. Eat only when you are genuinely hungry in your *stomach* and not in your imagination (when the hunger hormone *Ghrelin* indicates that your body needs 'fuel').
.
2. Eat slowly.

3. Stop eating when your stomach signals that it is *full* (when *Leptin* is released to indicate that your body has had enough 'fuel').</td></tr>
<tr><td>Breakfast</td><td>Did you have a healthy filling breakfast?
Yes ( ) No ( )</td></tr>
<tr><td>Mid-morning snack</td><td>Are you tummy hungry?
Do you need to eat?
Yes ( ) No ( )</td></tr>
<tr><td>Lunch</td><td>Did you follow the 'Three Point Plan'?
Yes ( ) No ( )</td></tr>
<tr><td>Mid-afternoon snack</td><td>Are you tummy hungry?
Do you need to eat?
Yes ( ) No ( )</td></tr>
<tr><td>Evening meal</td><td>Did you follow the 'Three Point Plan'?
Yes ( ) No ( )</td></tr>
<tr><td>Snack: watching TV movie, etc.,</td><td>Are you tummy hungry?
Do you need to eat?
Yes ( ) No ( )</td></tr>
<tr><td>Bedtime snack / supper</td><td>Are you tummy hungry?
Do you need to eat?
Yes ( ) No ( )</td></tr>
</table>

Exercise: Did you do something to make your heart beat faster?
Walking ( ) Other ( )

Foundation Phase 2
Week 3

Day 4 **Date** ________

Follow the 'Three Point Plan'.

1. Eat only when you are genuinely hungry in your *stomach* and not in your imagination (when the hunger hormone *Ghrelin* indicates that your body needs 'fuel').

.

2. Eat slowly.

3. Stop eating when your stomach signals that it is *full* (when *Leptin* is released to indicate that your body has had enough 'fuel').

Breakfast	Did you have a healthy filling breakfast? Yes ( ) No ( )
Mid-morning snack	Are you tummy hungry? Do you need to eat? Yes ( ) No ( )
Lunch	Did you follow the 'Three Point Plan'? Yes ( ) No ( )
Mid-afternoon snack	Are you tummy hungry? Do you need to eat? Yes ( ) No ( )
Evening meal	Did you follow the 'Three Point Plan'? Yes ( ) No ( )
Snack: watching TV movie, etc.,	Are you tummy hungry? Do you need to eat? Yes ( ) No ( )
Bedtime snack / supper	Are you tummy hungry? Do you need to eat? Yes ( ) No ( )

Exercise: Did you do something to make your heart beat faster?
Walking ( ) Other ( )

Foundation Phase 2
Week 3

Day 5 **Date** ________

Follow the 'Three Point Plan'.

1. Eat only when you are genuinely hungry in your *stomach* and not in your imagination (when the hunger hormone *Ghrelin* indicates that your body needs 'fuel').

.

2. Eat slowly.

3. Stop eating when your stomach signals that it is *full* (when *Leptin* is released to indicate that your body has had enough 'fuel').

Breakfast	Did you have a healthy filling breakfast? Yes ( ) No ( )
Mid-morning snack	Are you tummy hungry? Do you need to eat? Yes ( ) No ( )
Lunch	Did you follow the 'Three Point Plan'? Yes ( ) No ( )
Mid-afternoon snack	Are you tummy hungry? Do you need to eat? Yes ( ) No ( )
Evening meal	Did you follow the 'Three Point Plan'? Yes ( ) No ( )
Snack: watching TV movie, etc.,	Are you tummy hungry? Do you need to eat? Yes ( ) No ( )
Bedtime snack / supper	Are you tummy hungry? Do you need to eat? Yes ( ) No ( )

Exercise: Did you do something to make your heart beat faster?
Walking ( ) Other ( )

Foundation Phase 2
Week 3

Day 6 **Date ________**

'Treat Day'

Eat whatever you want and enjoy.

As you continue to follow this plan, you will find that you will gradually change the amount of 'treat' foods you eat.

Day 7 **Date ________**

In-between 'balance' day.

You will try to balance between following the 'Three Point Plan' and eating whatever you want and enjoy.

As you continue to follow this plan, you will find that you will gradually change the amount of 'treat' foods you eat.

Please keep faith in the plan.

Keep going and you will see real results.

Please complete the 'Review and progress check' on the next page.

Foundation Phase 2
Week 3

Day 7 **Date ________**

Review day and progress check.

Today is the day that you will stand on the scales and review your progress.

To achieve the most accurate weight, I suggest that you follow the procedure stated below.

- Weigh yourself first thing in the morning before breakfast.
- Wear as few clothes as possible (if any).
- Make sure the scales are set at zero.
- Stand on the correct part of the scale – see the manufacturer's instructions if you are not sure.
- Take three readings – they should all be the same. If you do get different readings, make sure that the scale is reset to zero before each reading.
- Write down the answer.
- Be honest and write down the true weight reading, not what you want the scales to say.

You may find it helpful to record the result below.

Weight: ______________

Weight lost: _____________

Did you lose any weight? Yes ( ) No ( )

If **yes**: well done and keep up the good work. You are re-educating your eating habits and are well on the way to achieving your weight loss goals.

Remember, you should aim to lose between 1 – 2 pounds per week.

If **no**: don't be discouraged. Ask yourself why - did you really follow the 'Three Point Plan' required for natural weight loss?

I know from my personal experience of following this plan that you can lose weight if you stick to the requirements of the programme. Start to follow the programme again and you should lose weight – if you follow the plan!

Well done!

You have completed *Phase 2* of the foundation stage of your weight loss journey.

It is now time to build upon your success in the first two phases. You shall now continue to establish the eating habits required to help you achieve and maintain your ideal natural weight.

Chapter 24

Daily programme: Foundation stage *Phase 3*

Change eating habits Support Plan & Progress tracker

This part of the plan builds upon Phase 1 & Phase 2 and follows a similar structure. The only difference in this phase is you can now start to think more seriously about 'Level B' exercise programmes in addition to your 'Level A' exercise. However, this is not essential at this stage.

Day 1 – 5 (Monday – Friday*): Main programme

Day 6: Treat day.

Day 7: In-between 'balance' day.

*If you work shift patterns which involve weekend work – no problem. Fit the 5 day support plan into your weekly schedule.

Please have faith in the plan and keep going - you will see results. It will take time, but it will be worth it as the weight loss will be real, natural and permanent.

Don't forget: You should make sure that you do some 'Level A' exercise every day. Also, you could start to think about doing some 'Level B' exercise programmes in addition to the on-going 'Level A' exercise.

Foundation Phase 3
Week 1

Day 1 **Date** ________

<table>
<tr><td colspan="2">Follow the 'Three Point Plan'.

1. Eat only when you are genuinely hungry in your *stomach* and not in your imagination (when the hunger hormone *Ghrelin* indicates that your body needs 'fuel').
.
2. Eat slowly.

3. Stop eating when your stomach signals that it is *full* (when *Leptin* is released to indicate that your body has had enough 'fuel').</td></tr>
<tr><td>Breakfast</td><td>Did you have a healthy filling breakfast?
Yes ( ) No ( )</td></tr>
<tr><td>Mid-morning snack</td><td>Are you tummy hungry?
Do you need to eat?
Yes ( ) No ( )</td></tr>
<tr><td>Lunch</td><td>Did you follow the 'Three Point Plan'?
Yes ( ) No ( )</td></tr>
<tr><td>Mid-afternoon snack</td><td>Are you tummy hungry?
Do you need to eat?
Yes ( ) No ( )</td></tr>
<tr><td>Evening meal</td><td>Did you follow the 'Three Point Plan'?
Yes ( ) No ( )</td></tr>
<tr><td>Snack: watching TV movie, etc.,</td><td>Are you tummy hungry?
Do you need to eat?
Yes ( ) No ( )</td></tr>
<tr><td>Bedtime snack / supper</td><td>Are you tummy hungry?
Do you need to eat?
Yes ( ) No ( )</td></tr>
</table>

Exercise: Did you do something to make your heart beat faster?
Walking ( ) Other ( )

Foundation Phase 3
Week 1

Day 2 **Date ________**

Follow the 'Three Point Plan'.

1. Eat only when you are genuinely hungry in your *stomach* and not in your imagination (when the hunger hormone *Ghrelin* indicates that your body needs 'fuel').

.

2. Eat slowly.

3. Stop eating when your stomach signals that it is *full* (when *Leptin* is released to indicate that your body has had enough 'fuel').

Breakfast	Did you have a healthy filling breakfast? Yes ( ) No ( )
Mid-morning snack	Are you tummy hungry? Do you need to eat? Yes ( ) No ( )
Lunch	Did you follow the 'Three Point Plan'? Yes ( ) No ( )
Mid-afternoon snack	Are you tummy hungry? Do you need to eat? Yes ( ) No ( )
Evening meal	Did you follow the 'Three Point Plan'? Yes ( ) No ( )
Snack: watching TV movie, etc.,	Are you tummy hungry? Do you need to eat? Yes ( ) No ( )
Bedtime snack / supper	Are you tummy hungry? Do you need to eat? Yes ( ) No ( )

Exercise: Did you do something to make your heart beat faster?
Walking ( ) Other ( )

Foundation Phase 3
Week 1

Day 3 **Date** ________

<table>
<tr><td colspan="2">Follow the 'Three Point Plan'.

1. Eat only when you are genuinely hungry in your *stomach* and not in your imagination (when the hunger hormone *Ghrelin* indicates that your body needs 'fuel').
.
2. Eat slowly.

3. Stop eating when your stomach signals that it is *full* (when *Leptin* is released to indicate that your body has had enough 'fuel').</td></tr>
<tr><td>Breakfast</td><td>Did you have a healthy filling breakfast?
Yes ( ) No ( )</td></tr>
<tr><td>Mid-morning snack</td><td>Are you tummy hungry?
Do you need to eat?
Yes ( ) No ( )</td></tr>
<tr><td>Lunch</td><td>Did you follow the 'Three Point Plan'?
Yes ( ) No ( )</td></tr>
<tr><td>Mid-afternoon snack</td><td>Are you tummy hungry?
Do you need to eat?
Yes ( ) No ( )</td></tr>
<tr><td>Evening meal</td><td>Did you follow the 'Three Point Plan'?
Yes ( ) No ( )</td></tr>
<tr><td>Snack: watching TV movie, etc.,</td><td>Are you tummy hungry?
Do you need to eat?
Yes ( ) No ( )</td></tr>
<tr><td>Bedtime snack / supper</td><td>Are you tummy hungry?
Do you need to eat?
Yes ( ) No ( )</td></tr>
</table>

Exercise: Did you do something to make your heart beat faster?
Walking ( ) Other ( )

Foundation Phase 3
Week 1

Day 4 **Date ________**

Follow the 'Three Point Plan'. **1. Eat only when you are genuinely hungry in your *stomach* and not in your imagination** (when the hunger hormone *Ghrelin* indicates that your body needs 'fuel'). . **2. Eat slowly.** **3. Stop eating when your stomach signals that it is *full*** (when *Leptin* is released to indicate that your body has had enough 'fuel').	
Breakfast	Did you have a healthy filling breakfast? Yes ( ) No ( )
Mid-morning snack	Are you tummy hungry? Do you need to eat? Yes ( ) No ( )
Lunch	Did you follow the 'Three Point Plan'? Yes ( ) No ( )
Mid-afternoon snack	Are you tummy hungry? Do you need to eat? Yes ( ) No ( )
Evening meal	Did you follow the 'Three Point Plan'? Yes ( ) No ( )
Snack: watching TV movie, etc.,	Are you tummy hungry? Do you need to eat? Yes ( ) No ( )
Bedtime snack / supper	Are you tummy hungry? Do you need to eat? Yes ( ) No ( )

Exercise: Did you do something to make your heart beat faster?
Walking ( ) Other ( )

Foundation Phase 3
Week 1

Day 5 **Date ________**

<table>
<tr><td colspan="2">Follow the 'Three Point Plan'.

1. Eat only when you are genuinely hungry in your stomach and not in your imagination (when the hunger hormone Ghrelin indicates that your body needs 'fuel').
.
2. Eat slowly.

3. Stop eating when your stomach signals that it is full (when Leptin is released to indicate that your body has had enough 'fuel').</td></tr>
<tr><td>Breakfast</td><td>Did you have a healthy filling breakfast?
Yes ( ) No ( )</td></tr>
<tr><td>Mid-morning snack</td><td>Are you tummy hungry?
Do you need to eat?
Yes ( ) No ( )</td></tr>
<tr><td>Lunch</td><td>Did you follow the 'Three Point Plan'?
Yes ( ) No ( )</td></tr>
<tr><td>Mid-afternoon snack</td><td>Are you tummy hungry?
Do you need to eat?
Yes ( ) No ( )</td></tr>
<tr><td>Evening meal</td><td>Did you follow the 'Three Point Plan'?
Yes ( ) No ( )</td></tr>
<tr><td>Snack: watching TV movie, etc.,</td><td>Are you tummy hungry?
Do you need to eat?
Yes ( ) No ( )</td></tr>
<tr><td>Bedtime snack / supper</td><td>Are you tummy hungry?
Do you need to eat?
Yes ( ) No ( )</td></tr>
</table>

Exercise: Did you do something to make your heart beat faster?
Walking ( ) Other ( )

Foundation Phase 3
Week 1

Day 6 **Date ________**

'Treat Day'

Eat whatever you want and enjoy.

As you continue to follow this plan, you will find that you will gradually change the amount of 'treat' foods you eat.

Day 7 **Date ________**

In-between 'balance' day.

You will try to balance between following the 'Three Point Plan' and eating whatever you want and enjoy.

As you continue to follow this plan, you will find that you will gradually change the amount of 'treat' foods you eat.

Please keep faith in the plan.

Keep going and you will see real results.

Foundation Phase 3
Week 2

Day 1 **Date ________**

Follow the 'Three Point Plan'.

1. Eat only when you are genuinely hungry in your *stomach* and not in your imagination (when the hunger hormone *Ghrelin* indicates that your body needs 'fuel').

.

2. Eat slowly.

3. Stop eating when your stomach signals that it is *full* (when *Leptin* is released to indicate that your body has had enough 'fuel').

Breakfast	Did you have a healthy filling breakfast? Yes ( ) No ( )
Mid-morning snack	Are you tummy hungry? Do you need to eat? Yes ( ) No ( )
Lunch	Did you follow the 'Three Point Plan'? Yes ( ) No ( )
Mid-afternoon snack	Are you tummy hungry? Do you need to eat? Yes ( ) No ( )
Evening meal	Did you follow the 'Three Point Plan'? Yes ( ) No ( )
Snack: watching TV movie, etc.,	Are you tummy hungry? Do you need to eat? Yes ( ) No ( )
Bedtime snack / supper	Are you tummy hungry? Do you need to eat? Yes ( ) No ( )

Exercise: Did you do something to make your heart beat faster?
Walking ( ) Other ( )

Foundation Phase 3
Week 2

Day 2 **Date ________**

<table>
<tr><td colspan="2">Follow the 'Three Point Plan'.

1. Eat only when you are genuinely hungry in your *stomach* and not in your imagination (when the hunger hormone *Ghrelin* indicates that your body needs 'fuel').
.
2. Eat slowly.

3. Stop eating when your stomach signals that it is *full* (when *Leptin* is released to indicate that your body has had enough 'fuel').</td></tr>
<tr><td>Breakfast</td><td>Did you have a healthy filling breakfast?
Yes ( ) No ( )</td></tr>
<tr><td>Mid-morning snack</td><td>Are you tummy hungry?
Do you need to eat?
Yes ( ) No ( )</td></tr>
<tr><td>Lunch</td><td>Did you follow the 'Three Point Plan'?
Yes ( ) No ( )</td></tr>
<tr><td>Mid-afternoon snack</td><td>Are you tummy hungry?
Do you need to eat?
Yes ( ) No ( )</td></tr>
<tr><td>Evening meal</td><td>Did you follow the 'Three Point Plan'?
Yes ( ) No ( )</td></tr>
<tr><td>Snack: watching TV movie, etc.,</td><td>Are you tummy hungry?
Do you need to eat?
Yes ( ) No ( )</td></tr>
<tr><td>Bedtime snack / supper</td><td>Are you tummy hungry?
Do you need to eat?
Yes ( ) No ( )</td></tr>
</table>

Exercise: Did you do something to make your heart beat faster?
Walking ( ) Other ( )

Foundation Phase 3
Week 2

Day 3 **Date ________**

Follow the 'Three Point Plan'. **1. Eat only when you are genuinely hungry in your *stomach* and not in your imagination** (when the hunger hormone *Ghrelin* indicates that your body needs 'fuel'). . **2. Eat slowly.** **3. Stop eating when your stomach signals that it is *full*** (when *Leptin* is released to indicate that your body has had enough 'fuel').	
Breakfast	Did you have a healthy filling breakfast? Yes ( ) No ( )
Mid-morning snack	Are you tummy hungry? Do you need to eat? Yes ( ) No ( )
Lunch	Did you follow the 'Three Point Plan'? Yes ( ) No ( )
Mid-afternoon snack	Are you tummy hungry? Do you need to eat? Yes ( ) No ( )
Evening meal	Did you follow the 'Three Point Plan'? Yes ( ) No ( )
Snack: watching TV movie, etc.,	Are you tummy hungry? Do you need to eat? Yes ( ) No ( )
Bedtime snack / supper	Are you tummy hungry? Do you need to eat? Yes ( ) No ( )

Exercise: Did you do something to make your heart beat faster?
Walking ( ) Other ( )

Foundation Phase 3
Week 2

Day 4 **Date ________**

<table>
<tr><td colspan="2">Follow the 'Three Point Plan'.

1. Eat only when you are genuinely hungry in your stomach and not in your imagination (when the hunger hormone Ghrelin indicates that your body needs 'fuel').
.
2. Eat slowly.

3. Stop eating when your stomach signals that it is full (when Leptin is released to indicate that your body has had enough 'fuel').</td></tr>
<tr><td>Breakfast</td><td>Did you have a healthy filling breakfast?
Yes ( ) No ( )</td></tr>
<tr><td>Mid-morning snack</td><td>Are you tummy hungry?
Do you need to eat?
Yes ( ) No ( )</td></tr>
<tr><td>Lunch</td><td>Did you follow the 'Three Point Plan'?
Yes ( ) No ( )</td></tr>
<tr><td>Mid-afternoon snack</td><td>Are you tummy hungry?
Do you need to eat?
Yes ( ) No ( )</td></tr>
<tr><td>Evening meal</td><td>Did you follow the 'Three Point Plan'?
Yes ( ) No ( )</td></tr>
<tr><td>Snack: watching TV movie, etc.,</td><td>Are you tummy hungry?
Do you need to eat?
Yes ( ) No ( )</td></tr>
<tr><td>Bedtime snack / supper</td><td>Are you tummy hungry?
Do you need to eat?
Yes ( ) No ( )</td></tr>
</table>

Exercise: Did you do something to make your heart beat faster?
Walking ( ) Other ( )

Foundation Phase 3
Week 2

Day 5 **Date ________**

Follow the 'Three Point Plan'.

1. Eat only when you are genuinely hungry in your *stomach* and not in your imagination (when the hunger hormone *Ghrelin* indicates that your body needs 'fuel').

.

2. Eat slowly.

3. Stop eating when your stomach signals that it is *full* (when *Leptin* is released to indicate that your body has had enough 'fuel').

Breakfast	Did you have a healthy filling breakfast? Yes ( ) No ( )
Mid-morning snack	Are you tummy hungry? Do you need to eat? Yes ( ) No ( )
Lunch	Did you follow the 'Three Point Plan'? Yes ( ) No ( )
Mid-afternoon snack	Are you tummy hungry? Do you need to eat? Yes ( ) No ( )
Evening meal	Did you follow the 'Three Point Plan'? Yes ( ) No ( )
Snack: watching TV movie, etc.,	Are you tummy hungry? Do you need to eat? Yes ( ) No ( )
Bedtime snack / supper	Are you tummy hungry? Do you need to eat? Yes ( ) No ( )

Exercise: Did you do something to make your heart beat faster?
Walking ( ) Other ( )

Foundation Phase 3
Week 2

Day 6 **Date ________**

'Treat Day'

Eat whatever you want and enjoy.

As you continue to follow this plan, you will find that you will gradually change the amount of 'treat' foods you eat.

Day 7 **Date ________**

In-between 'balance' day.

You will try to balance between following the 'Three Point Plan' and eating whatever you want and enjoy.

As you continue to follow this plan, you will find that you will gradually change the amount of 'treat' foods you eat.

Please keep faith in the plan.

Keep going and you will see real results.

Foundation Phase 3
Week 3

Day 1 **Date ________**

Follow the 'Three Point Plan'. **1. Eat only when you are genuinely hungry in your *stomach* and not in your imagination** (when the hunger hormone *Ghrelin* indicates that your body needs 'fuel'). . **2. Eat slowly.** **3. Stop eating when your stomach signals that it is *full*** (when *Leptin* is released to indicate that your body has had enough 'fuel').	
Breakfast	Did you have a healthy filling breakfast? Yes ( ) No ( )
Mid-morning snack	Are you tummy hungry? Do you need to eat? Yes ( ) No ( )
Lunch	Did you follow the 'Three Point Plan'? Yes ( ) No ( )
Mid-afternoon snack	Are you tummy hungry? Do you need to eat? Yes ( ) No ( )
Evening meal	Did you follow the 'Three Point Plan'? Yes ( ) No ( )
Snack: watching TV movie, etc.,	Are you tummy hungry? Do you need to eat? Yes ( ) No ( )
Bedtime snack / supper	Are you tummy hungry? Do you need to eat? Yes ( ) No ( )

Exercise: Did you do something to make your heart beat faster?
Walking ( ) Other ( )

Foundation Phase 3
Week 3

Day 2 **Date** ________

Follow the 'Three Point Plan'. **1. Eat only when you are genuinely hungry in your *stomach* and not in your imagination** (when the hunger hormone *Ghrelin* indicates that your body needs 'fuel'). . **2. Eat slowly.** **3. Stop eating when your stomach signals that it is *full*** (when *Leptin* is released to indicate that your body has had enough 'fuel').	
Breakfast	Did you have a healthy filling breakfast? Yes ( ) No ( )
Mid-morning snack	Are you tummy hungry? Do you need to eat? Yes ( ) No ( )
Lunch	Did you follow the 'Three Point Plan'? Yes ( ) No ( )
Mid-afternoon snack	Are you tummy hungry? Do you need to eat? Yes ( ) No ( )
Evening meal	Did you follow the 'Three Point Plan'? Yes ( ) No ( )
Snack: watching TV movie, etc.,	Are you tummy hungry? Do you need to eat? Yes ( ) No ( )
Bedtime snack / supper	Are you tummy hungry? Do you need to eat? Yes ( ) No ( )

Exercise: Did you do something to make your heart beat faster?
Walking ( ) Other ( )

Foundation Phase 3
Week 3

Day 3 **Date ________**

Follow the 'Three Point Plan'.

1. Eat only when you are genuinely hungry in your *stomach* and not in your imagination (when the hunger hormone *Ghrelin* indicates that your body needs 'fuel').

.

2. Eat slowly.

3. Stop eating when your stomach signals that it is *full* (when *Leptin* is released to indicate that your body has had enough 'fuel').

Breakfast	Did you have a healthy filling breakfast? Yes ( ) No ( )
Mid-morning snack	Are you tummy hungry? Do you need to eat? Yes ( ) No ( )
Lunch	Did you follow the 'Three Point Plan'? Yes ( ) No ( )
Mid-afternoon snack	Are you tummy hungry? Do you need to eat? Yes ( ) No ( )
Evening meal	Did you follow the 'Three Point Plan'? Yes ( ) No ( )
Snack: watching TV movie, etc.,	Are you tummy hungry? Do you need to eat? Yes ( ) No ( )
Bedtime snack / supper	Are you tummy hungry? Do you need to eat? Yes ( ) No ( )

Exercise: Did you do something to make your heart beat faster?
Walking ( ) Other ( )

Foundation Phase 3
Week 3

Day 4 **Date ________**

Follow the 'Three Point Plan'.

1. Eat only when you are genuinely hungry in your *stomach* and not in your imagination (when the hunger hormone *Ghrelin* indicates that your body needs 'fuel').

.

2. Eat slowly.

3. Stop eating when your stomach signals that it is *full* (when *Leptin* is released to indicate that your body has had enough 'fuel').

Breakfast	Did you have a healthy filling breakfast? Yes ( ) No ( )
Mid-morning snack	Are you tummy hungry? Do you need to eat? Yes ( ) No ( )
Lunch	Did you follow the 'Three Point Plan'? Yes ( ) No ( )
Mid-afternoon snack	Are you tummy hungry? Do you need to eat? Yes ( ) No ( )
Evening meal	Did you follow the 'Three Point Plan'? Yes ( ) No ( )
Snack: watching TV movie, etc.,	Are you tummy hungry? Do you need to eat? Yes ( ) No ( )
Bedtime snack / supper	Are you tummy hungry? Do you need to eat? Yes ( ) No ( )

Exercise: Did you do something to make your heart beat faster?
Walking ( ) Other ( )

Foundation Phase 3
Week 3

Day 5 **Date ________**

Follow the 'Three Point Plan'. **1. Eat only when you are genuinely hungry in your *stomach* and not in your imagination** (when the hunger hormone *Ghrelin* indicates that your body needs 'fuel'). . **2. Eat slowly.** **3. Stop eating when your stomach signals that it is *full*** (when *Leptin* is released to indicate that your body has had enough 'fuel').	
Breakfast	Did you have a healthy filling breakfast? Yes ( ) No ( )
Mid-morning snack	Are you tummy hungry? Do you need to eat? Yes ( ) No ( )
Lunch	Did you follow the 'Three Point Plan'? Yes ( ) No ( )
Mid-afternoon snack	Are you tummy hungry? Do you need to eat? Yes ( ) No ( )
Evening meal	Did you follow the 'Three Point Plan'? Yes ( ) No ( )
Snack: watching TV movie, etc.,	Are you tummy hungry? Do you need to eat? Yes ( ) No ( )
Bedtime snack / supper	Are you tummy hungry? Do you need to eat? Yes ( ) No ( )

Exercise: Did you do something to make your heart beat faster?
Walking ( ) Other ( )

Foundation Phase 3
Week 3

Day 6 **Date ________**

'Treat Day'

Eat whatever you want and enjoy.

As you continue to follow this plan, you will find that you will gradually change the amount of 'treat' foods you eat.

Day 7 **Date ________**

In-between 'balance' day.

You will try to balance between following the 'Three Point Plan' and eating whatever you want and enjoy.

As you continue to follow this plan, you will find that you will gradually change the amount of 'treat' foods you eat.

Please keep faith in the plan.

Keep going and you will see real results.

Please complete the 'Review and progress check' on the next page.

Foundation Phase 2
Week 3

Day 7 **Date ________**

Review day and progress check.

Today is the day that you will stand on the scales and review your progress.

To achieve the most accurate weight, I suggest that you follow the procedure stated below.

- Weigh yourself first thing in the morning before breakfast.
- Wear as few clothes as possible (if any).
- Make sure the scales are set at zero.
- Stand on the correct part of the scale – see the manufacturer's instructions if you are not sure.
- Take three readings – they should all be the same. If you do get different readings, make sure that the scale is reset to zero before each reading.
- Write down the answer.
- Be honest and write down the true weight reading, not what you want the scales to say.

You may find it helpful to record the result below.

Weight: _____________

Weight lost: ____________

Did you lose any weight? Yes ( ) No ( )

If **yes**: well done and keep up the good work. You are re-educating your eating habits and are well on the way to achieving your weight loss goals.

Remember, you should aim to lose between 1 – 2 pounds per week.

If **no**: don't be discouraged. Ask yourself why - did you really follow the 'Three Point Plan' required for natural weight loss?

I know from my personal experience of following this plan that you can lose weight if you stick to the requirements of the programme. Start to follow the programme again from and you should lose weight – if you follow the plan!

Well done!

You have completed *Phase 3* of the foundation stage of your weight loss journey.

It is now time to build upon your success in the three foundation phases. You shall now continue to establish the eating habits required to help you achieve and maintain your ideal natural weight.

Chapter 25

The next phase – the rest of your life!

If you have followed the programme and used the 'Three Point Plan' as the tool to re-educate your eating habits, you will have put in place the foundation upon which you will now build your new eating habits.

You should have lost some weight by now – *if you have been following the principles of the 'Three Point Plan'.*

If you didn't lose weight.

If you have not lost any weight, it is time to be honest with yourself and review if you really did stick to the principles of the plan.

Please don't worry if this is the case, as the good news is you can always start again or pick up from where you left off.

It may take more than one attempt to establish the new eating habits being advocated by this book.

It is vital that you keep positive and have faith in yourself and the plan.

'If at first you don't succeed, try, try, try again'.

What next?

Continue to follow the 'Three Point Plan'.

Eventually you should follow these principles without thinking.

Start to think about the type of food items you eat.

You have laid the foundation regarding ***how*** you should eat, and established the good natural eating habits required to maintain your ideal healthy weight.

Now it is time to review ***what*** you eat. Think about healthy options and alternatives where appropriate.

Engage in some sort of appropriate 'Level B' exercise programme.

You should be engaging in 'Level A' exercise activities as a natural part of you daily life and routine.

It is time to start to think seriously about which 'Level B' programmes you would like to engage in.

Final thoughts

I would like to offer you my best wishes as you continue on your journey to achieve and maintain the ideal weight, health and fitness levels you are looking for.

It will not always be easy, especially during the early stages; however, following the natural weight loss principles outlined in this book is actually much easier than 'going on a diet'.

Furthermore, the weight loss achieved by following the '*Three Point Plan*' (in contrast 'dieting') should be gradual but *permanent* – if you stick to the principles of the plan!

The effectiveness of this approach to weight management has been proven by my own experience.

If I can do it – so can you!

www.ingramcontent.com/pod-product-compliance
Lightning Source LLC
Chambersburg PA
CBHW050112280326
41933CB00010B/1071
* 9 7 8 0 9 9 5 4 9 0 6 2 8 *